Recent Health Policy Innovations in Social Security

T0386509

International Social Security Series

In cooperation with the
International Social Security Association (ISSA)
Neil Gilbert, Series Editor

Recent Health Policy Innovations in Social Security

Edited by

Aviva Ron
Xenia Scheil-Adlung

International Social Security Series
Volume 5

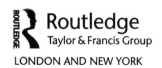

Routledge
Taylor & Francis Group

LONDON AND NEW YORK

The International Social Security Association (ISSA) was founded in 1927. It is a non-profit international organization bringing together institutions and administrative bodies from countries all over the world dealing with all forms of compulsory social protection. The objective of the ISSA is to cooperate at the international level, in the promotion and development of social security throughout the world, primarily by improving techniques and administration in order to advance people's social and economic conditions on the basis of social justice.

First published 2001 by Transaction Publishers

Published 2017 by Routledge
2 Park Square, Milton Park, Abingdon, Oxon OX14 4RN
711 Third Avenue, New York, NY 10017, USA

Routledge is an imprint of the Taylor & Francis Group, an informa business

Library of Congress Catalog Number: 00-054382

Library of Congress Cataloging-in-Publication Data

Recent health policy innovations in social security / edited by Aviva Ron, Xenia Scheil-Adlung
    p. cm.— (International social security series ; v. 5)
    Includes bibliographical references and index.
    ISBN 0-7658-0753-X (alk. paper)
    1. Medicine, State. 2. Insurance, health. 3. Medical care, Cost of. 4. Health care reform. I. Ron, Aviva. II. Scheil-Adlung, Xenia. III. Series.

RA411 .R434 2001
362.1—dc21   00-054382

ISBN 13: 978-0-7658-0753-3 (pbk)

Contents

Part 1

Introduction

1

Worldwide Innovations in Health Insurance Reform

X. Scheil-Adlung

In most countries today social health insurance forms an important part of daily life for the population and is regarded as extremely important. However, systems that have developed gradually over many years now find themselves confronted by clearly defined limits. There are still population sectors excluded from social protection without equal access to health insurance. Severe funding problems and cost increases set limits on possibilities for reform and population ageing is leading to new pressures on costs.

- How can adequate health care be provided for as many people as possible at reasonable contributions and cost?

- How can funding shortfalls, over- and under-provision of care, waste and administrative inefficiency in social health insurance systems be prevented?

- How can health care institutions be organized in a more future-oriented way?

- What solutions are there to such structural problems for health insurance systems with population ageing and its concomitant upward pressure on costs?

Both industrialized and developing countries have been working intensively for several years on answers to these central questions for social health insurance systems.

How can adequate health care be provided for as many people as possible at a reasonable cost?

The search for solutions with regard to more equal access to health care involves both the formal and informal sectors of the economy. Efforts are aimed in particular at social health insurance for salaried workers, the self-employed, immigrants, asylum seekers, illegal workers, domestic and agricultural workers, and family dependents.

How can funding shortfalls, over- and under-provision of care, waste and administrative inefficiency in social health care systems be prevented?

Most countries are being forced to look for new, socially acceptable solutions as a result of rising financial pressure on state budgets and rising health costs.

- In statistical terms[1] the 1994 figures for per-capita expenditure on health varied from US$1,196 in Southeast Asia and the Pacific and up to US$21,169 in established market economies. For the same period health spending as a percentage of

Table 1.1
Health Care Spending by Region, 1994

Region	Per-capita spending in US$	Health care spending as a percentage of GDP	Percentage of public expenditure on health care
Asia and the Pacific (incl. China)	1,196	3.9	53
Eastern Europe and Central Asia	3,847	6.3	69
Latin America and the Caribbean	5,801	6	56
Middle East and North Africa	7,181	4.6	53
Southern Asia (incl. India)	1,887	3.5	44
Sub-Sahara	2,070	4.1	51
Established market economies	21,169	8.3	77

Source: Adapted from G. Schieber; A. Maeda. 1997. "A Curmudgeon's guide to financing health care in developing countries," World Bank, An International Conference, *Innovations in health care financing*," Washington D.C., March 10-11.

GDP varied from less than 4 percent (Southeast Asia and the Pacific) to over 8 percent (established market economies). The public share of health spending varied from 44 percent (Southeast Asia including India) to 77 percent (established market economies) as table 1.1 shows.

On the one hand financial pressures lead to the search for new funding sources and methods, while on the other the possibilities for rationalization have largely been exhausted. Efforts are now being directed at removing over- and under-provision of health care and administrative inefficiency and using new information technology to provide better services.

The pressures of costs, however, are also leading to a situation where a delicate balance between the affordable, and the socially desirable has to be found and defended politically. Each decision is of great ethical importance. In the final analysis the extent of health care provided decides who lives or survives, to what extent people live in pain and suffering, and who dies.[2]

How can social health insurance institutions be organized in a more future-oriented way?

The question about organizing social health insurance systems in a more future-oriented way is central to the problem of a balanced relationship between the public and private sectors, or mixed approaches between the two, such as mutual benefit societies. Profit- or non-profit-oriented institutions that are public or private can exist alongside non-profit-oriented public institutions which provide health services. The deciding factor in all cases should be the extent to which such approaches positively influence efficiency and health care provision for the population.

What solutions lead the way out of structural problems for health insurance systems, such as population ageing and associated pressures on costs?

It is becoming increasingly clear in many countries that health insurance systems will have to focus benefits more tightly on the needs of the population. This is particularly true for sectors such as prevention, rehabilitation, primary care and long-term care for an ageing population. Many systems show deficits in these areas, which ultimately lead to increased costs.

The results of the reform debate, which has gone on for many years in some cases, about the questions raised above often contain innovative ideas for reform that could transcend national boundaries. The debate sees great opportunities in

- a future-oriented extension of health insurance with the framework of social protection;

- a progressive development of funding methods;

- an appropriate exertion of influence on expenditure;

- bringing benefits into line with what is actually needed;

- the use of technological advances.

The aim of this publication is to present those important innovations to social health insurance systems in industrialized and developing countries that have been brought in over recent years and, as far as possible, already evaluated. In doing so, the intention is to show the developments that are valid for more than one country which could be relevant in the longer term for taking health insurance systems forward.

The International Social Security Association (ISSA) intends, with this publication, a deeper exchange of experience between differing regions, countries, and health insurance systems, thus providing ideas for politicians and practitioners, scientists, and other experts.

The publication will concentrate on innovations in health insurance policy in the areas mentioned above taken from selected countries in

- Africa, using Morocco and Zimbabwe as examples;

- America, using Uruguay and the United States, amongst others, as examples;

- Asia, particularly India, China, Japan and Vietnam;

- Europe, particularly France and Germany,

for presentation and analysis. In addition this publication will address recent institutional economic findings and selected questions with regard to information technology in health insurance systems from a fundamental point of view.

The publication is divided into six parts dealing with the following topics:

- *New approaches in extending coverage in a health insurance system*

Aviva Ron and Wouter van Ginneken report on new approaches to extending social protection against illness for those in work in formal and informal economic sectors. Both authors use examples from developing countries.

- *Confronting resource scarcity: Innovative strategies*

William Newbrander and Rena Eichler refer to the history, organization, and future of successful methods to limit costs through Managed Care in the United States. Aidi Hu presents in detail innovative aspects of health insurance in China combining the pro-rata approach with capital-based coverage.

- *Refining benefits to meet current needs*

Werner Müller-Fahrnow, Thomas Hansmeier, and Karla Spyra report on trends in benefits, which are characterized, among other things, by improved integration of prevention and rehabilitation programs. Xenia Scheil-Adlung and Naoki Iguchi present innovative solutions for those in need of long-term care from selected countries in Europe and Asia, and analyze the extent to which population trends are being overcome from the point of view of social health care systems.

- *New institutional and administrative frameworks*

What new institutional and administrative solutions have characterized trends in health care systems over recent years? Aviva Ron addresses basic issues here while Navin Girishankar, April Harding, and Alexander Preker present recent new findings from the institutional economic field and examine the changing role of the state in particular. Practical solutions from Africa, Europe and Latin America, using the example of mutual benefit societies, are presented by Maurice Duranton, Abdellatif Zuaq, and Julio Pilón.

- *Transformation through information technology systems*

Great importance is also attached to information technology systems in changing the field of health insurance. In particular these can be used to achieve improved efficiency and make use of any rationalization possibilities that remain. Claude Delaveau comments on the fundamental possibilities offered by information technology systems. Gerhard Brenner presents aims, requirements, barriers, and components in his contribution, while Bernd Blobel deals with the problems of data protection in detail.

Many of the innovations presented here have already been integrated into existing reforms and the authors refer to concrete developments in individual countries and regions. In order to give the reader the possibility of forming an opinion on innovative approaches in individual countries in a wider context, a brief overview follows of recent trends and reforms in selected health insurance systems in various regions, and covers innovations in both health care benefits and cash sickness allowances in the systems reviewed.

Recent Trends in Health Care Systems in Africa: The Introduction and Further Development of Statutory Insurance Schemes

Many African countries have set up their health care systems as insurance-based systems and established successful mutual benefit societies,[3] particularly in North Africa. The efforts directed at setting up health care systems throughout the rest of Africa can be characterized as *the introduction and further development of statutory insurance schemes.*

As shown in table 1.2, these efforts refer to the creation of health insurance schemes in Burundi, Kenya, Namibia, the Sudan, and South Africa.

The starting point for the reform efforts in almost all these countries in Africa was the wish for improved health care for the population through health care benefits and the desire to cope with the financial burden that these entailed through the insurance mechanism.

For example, in the Sudan, the absence of development aid and loans, together with rising health costs, led to a worsening in medical care provision. As a result the government decided on the gradual introduction of a new health insurance scheme covering employees and their dependents.

The newly introduced health insurance schemes in most countries were characterized by strong social elements pushing back the importance of private insurance schemes in some cases:

- For example, in Kenya, where statutory system coverage was met by private insurance schemes by up to 11.4 percent,[4] a national health insurance fund was planned to strengthen the feeling of solidarity and justice between various income groups, and improve access to care, and the quality of that care.

- In the Sudan free benefits for the poor were introduced together with state subsidies to finance the system.

- The health insurance reform in South Africa also aimed at finding solutions to help the poor. On the one hand, plans exist to introduce compensation funds between

Table 1.2
Selected Reforms for Social Protection against Sickness
in Africa, 1996-1998, by Country

Country	Health care system	Reform	Date of implementation
Burundi	Need-oriented medical care provision	Creation of a health insurance scheme	1996
Ivory Coast	Social insurance scheme	Introduction of a sickness cash allowance of up to six months	1996
Kenya	Social insurance scheme	Introduction of a national health insurance fund	By 2002
Namibia	-	Introduction of national funds for maternity benefits, sick leave and funeral allowances, as well as for health insurance	1995, 1998
Sudan	-	Introduction of a social health insurance scheme	1995, 2000
South Africa	Social insurance scheme	Introduction of basic medical care provision for the whole population	1996
		Introduction of a health insurance scheme to cover hospital charges	
Tunisia	Social insurance scheme	Changes in reimbursement levels	1996
		Benefit reduction for convalescent stays	

Sources: Social Security Administration, "Social security throughout the world," 1997, Washington DC, ISSA, Data Base "Developments and Trends"; Erika de Wet, "Reformtendenzen im südafrikanischen Gesundheits-und Krankenversicherungssystem: eine erste Bilanz," in *Zeitschrift für Sozialreform*, 8/1997, pp. 477-492.

health insurance schemes and a variety of risk structures in order to be able to guarantee basic medical care for the whole population. On the other hand, the disproportionate relationship between private and public medical care provision is to be remedied to some extent in South Africa in the future. Approximately 60 percent of all health expenditure is spent on the 23 percent of the population who are privately insured.[5] In future private care provision is also to be made available for the poor.

Financial reasons are at the center of far-reaching reforms in Tunisia. There are plans to involve those insured more in financial responsibility and to introduce cost sharing in stages. Here again, however, social criteria for the poor were taken into account. Cost sharing ceilings for expensive courses of treatment have been introduced in order not to restrict the right to benefit access.

Some countries, such as Benin, Guinea, Cameroon, and Nigeria, which have not carried out any fundamental reform of their health insurance systems, have been concentrating in recent years on basic medical care and achieving local improvements in quality. In these countries, currently only the formal salaried sector workers are covered.

Furthermore, attempts at extending health care coverage to those working in the formal and informal economic sectors are becoming increasingly widespread.[6]

Trends on the American Continent: Extending the Scope of Health Care Systems and Improving Efficiency

Just as in the case of Africa, common trends and focal points for reform efforts can be identified on the American continent over the period 1996 to 1998. These focal points are,

- extension of the scope of social protection in the case of illness; and

- improvements in institutional efficiency.

See table 1.3 for selected reforms with regard to social protection in the case of sickness in countries on the American continent.

Both in North and South America[7] the main efforts are directed at making better use of scarce resources in order to make medical benefits available to larger sectors of the population. In doing so a search is also taking place at the different financial and institutional levels for solutions that are better balanced in social terms than previously. The reforms in Peru and the United States serve as examples and details of these reforms are presented below.

Extending the scope

Efforts to extend the scope of coverage in Peru also include minimum and additional benefits for employees and other specified groups. A state health care system for persons on low incomes was also introduced, as can be seen from table 1.4.

Table 1. 3
Selected Reforms with Regard to Social Protection in the Case of Sickness in
America, 1996-1998, by Country

Country	Health care system	Reform	Date of implementation
El Salvador	Social insurance scheme	Introduction of a supplementary insurance scheme to children aged 5-6	1996
Mexico	Social insurance scheme	New regulations governing contributions Introduction of a family sickness insurance authority	1997
Peru	Social insurance scheme	Introduction of a 3-pillar health care system	1997
Saint Vincent and Grenada	Social insurance scheme and private insurance scheme	Acceptance of self-employed individuals into the insurance system	1997
United States	Social insurance scheme	Extension of health insurance coverage when changing employment Introduction of savings accounts for medical care Introduction of standards on the exchange of medical data	1996 1999, 2002

Sources: ISSA, Data Base "Developments and Trends," Jürgen Krause, *Das Krankenversicherungssystem der USA*, Baden-Baden, 1997, Nomos.

Table 1.4
Peru: Introduction of a 3-Pillar Health Care System

The Peruvian Congress has adopted a law which establishes a reformed health system divided into three main pillars.

The Social Health Scheme (Seguro Social de Salud [SSS])
The new scheme is to be managed by the *Instituto Peruano de Seguridad Social (IPSS)* and will cover two classes of members: ordinary members and voluntary members. Ordinary members, for whom coverage will be compulsory, will be active workers in a dependent employment relationship or associates of workers' cooperatives. People who are not eligible as ordinary members will be entitled to coverage as voluntary members. In addition, spouses, partners and dependent children will also be covered. A health plan is to be developed which will set out the minimum level of benefits and services to be provided to SSS members.

Complementary Health Plans and Programs
Complementary health plans and programs will be provided by public or private organizations. Employers will be able to use their own infrastructure, where available, or to contract licensed Health Service Organizations (Entidades Prestadoras de Salud [EPS]) to provide services under a complementary plan. Where an EPS is used, it is to be selected through a majority vote of employees. People will be able to join an EPS on a voluntary basis, and workers will also have the option of being covered by the State Health Services rather than using services provided by employers or EPS organizations.

The extent of the services provided by employers is to be independent of the income level of workers. These services must include the treatment of employment injuries and cannot exclude the treatment of pre-existing diseases.

State Health Service (Régimen Estatal de Salud)
The State Health Service will be an integrated service for people on low incomes who do not have access to other schemes. It will be administered by the Ministry of Health.

Administration of the New System
Supervision of the organizations providing health services will be the responsibility of the Superintendencia de Entidades Prestadoras de Salud (SEPS).

Financing of the Services
The services provided by the SSS will be financed from monthly contributions according to the type of membership. Co-payments for health services will also be required from complementary health plan members. Co-payments will not exceed a set percentage of a member's income.
Employers who provide services, either themselves or through an EPS, will be able to offset part of the corresponding costs from their contribution to the IPSS.

References: Decreto Legislativo núm. 887, Ley de Modernización de la Seguridad Social en Salud; Ley núm. 26790.

Source: Cuadernos laborales, vol. 16, núm. 119, 1996-1997 (ISSA Data Bank "Developments and Trends").

Table 1.5 shows that the focus on extending social protection in the case of sickness in the United States lies, on the one hand, in plugging gaps in the insurance coverage for employees when they change jobs and, on the other hand, in extending coverage to include those working for "small enterprises," and pensioners.

The efforts to extend coverage in the United States take the form of the introduction of "Medical Savings Accounts" aimed at (partially) financing medical benefits directly.

Medical Savings Accounts are accounts opened with, and administered by, institutions such as banks and insurance companies. The regulations governing them are similar to those for individual old-age provision schemes. These accounts and their revenue are tax-free.[8]

Reforms aimed at extending the scope of coverage to include additional sectors of the population (children and self-employed persons) were also introduced in El Salvador and Saint Vincent and Grenada.

In Mexico the scope of coverage was extended as part of institutional changes. The introduction of a new family insurance authority (*Seguro de Salud para la Familia*) is designed to make basic medical care available to those persons who are not members of the general Mexican Social Insurance Institute.

Improvements in Efficiency

Efforts to extend the scope of health insurance coverage often go hand in hand with efforts to improve efficiency in the health care systems concerned. Just as in Mexico, with the introduction of the family health insurance authority, Peru is also seeking increased efficiency through new institutional structures. The introduction of the 3-pillar system was chosen with this in mind. The three pillars are a social health system for employees, the voluntary complementary system, and the state health service.

The United States has long been working with care provision structures such as the Health Management Organization (HMO) and Managed Care, both of which are now coming into use in Europe. The central concern here is to achieve the best possible use of resources taking market forces into account.[9]

Further efforts to increase efficiency—aimed at significantly reducing costs, primarily by simplifying administrative procedures through the introduction of electronic data transfer for medical

Table 1.5
United States: Extension of Insurance Coverage and Increases in Efficiency

Over 37 million Americans are without health insurance coverage, a further 22 million are insufficiently insured. The reason for this lack, or inadequacy of, insurance coverage is often loss or change of employment. Another problem area is the rising cost of the American health care system. These aspects have been taken into account in a reform, known as the "lesser health insurance reform," which can be divided into four main components.

1. Improvement of portability, accessibility and renewability of health insurance cover
Whereas up to the present there was no regulation in respect of the portability of health insurance in the event of change of employment, the new regulations guarantee insurance cover by regulating access, portability and renewability of health insurances for workers and, to some extent, also for their dependents. Furthermore, private insurance providers may no longer exclude persons in respect of preexisting illnesses or genetic findings, provided that specific conditions are met.

2. Precautions against fraud and abuse
Fines and numerous other penalties have been devised to prevent fraud and abuse in the domain of health insurance.

3. Simplification of administrative procedures to reduce bureaucracy and administrative costs
Steps are to be taken so that Medicare and Medicaid will be more efficient and costs reduced. To this effect, in particular standards and demands are to be established in respect of electronic health data bases. Chief among these are data concerned with the establishment and loss of memberships, distraints, as well as receipts and authorizations.

4. Tax incentives to extend the categories of insured persons
With the introduction of the Medical Savings Accounts, the category of insured persons is to be extended to include employees of "small enterprises" and pensioners.

According to the new regulations, employer contributions paid into such savings accounts are tax deductible. The accounts can only cover medical benefits, not the costs of a health insurance policy.

Under the terms of the project, however, pensioners receive a flat rate from Medicare, with which they can buy a health insurance with a high level of cost sharing. The remaining amount of the flat rate is then to be deposited in the tax-free savings accounts.

References: Health Insurance Profitability and Accountability Act of 1996; Balance Budget Act of 1997.

Sources: Jürgen Kruse, "Entwicklung des Gesundheitswesens in den USA," in *Informationsdienst der Gesellschaft für Versicherungswissenschaft und -gestaltung*, Cologne, 1997, ISSA, Data Base Developments and Trends."

records—are being made in the United States. The aim is to create a data network that conforms to certain standards and requirements. Further savings in administrative costs are expected from reductions in the bureaucracy attached to Medicare and Medicaid.

Asia and the Pacific:
Reforms Aimed at Benefits, Financing, and
Extension of Coverage

Health care provision in the Asia and Pacific region covers a multiplicity of systems not found in other regions. Here one finds social insurance schemes, provident funds, mixed systems, and much more.

Table 1.6 shows a selection of reforms in the area of social protection in the case of illness which have been carried out in the Asia and Pacific region.

A detailed examination of reforms shows that the focus of further developments in social protection against illness in Asia and the Pacific lies in the following directions:

- extending benefits;

- adjusting funding regulations; and

- increased coverage for the poor under social protection programs against sickness.

The reforms in the Republic of Korea and India can serve as examples of these trends and developments.

Benefit Extension

In the Republic of Korea benefit extension covers the period for which benefits are granted in the first instance. Over the next two years this period will be extended by a further thirty days. This removes any time limit on benefits. The catalogue of benefits for costly treatments has also been extended.

Further benefit improvements in the Asia and Pacific region have been introduced in Australia with an extension of the benefit period.

The reform of the Japanese health system is particularly important. Increased demands made as the result of population ageing are being met with new solutions for the need for long-term care.[10]

Table 1.6

Selected Reforms for Social Protection in the Case of Illness in Asia and the Pacific, 1996-1998, by Country

Country	Health care system	Reform	Date of implementation
Australia	Social benefit and universal health care system	Extension of the period for sickness cash benefit	1997
		No transfer from unemploy-ment benefit to sickness benefit	1996
China	Care provision through employer programmes, social insurance scheme, medical savings plans	Introduction of community funds (insurance funds) and individual savings accounts in selected areas	1997
India	Social insurance scheme	Introduction of a health insurance scheme for the poor	1996, 1997
		Rise in contributions to cover a million new insured persons and increase in benefits	1997
Iran	Social insurance scheme	Benefits limited to the first three children	1996
Japan	Social insurance scheme	Higher contributions and additional payments	1997
		Introduction of a long-term care insurance scheme	2000
South Korea	Social insurance scheme	Extension of the period over which benefits can be drawn	1996
		New reimbursement system	1996
		Consolidation of insurance funds	
Singapore	Employer programme, Provident Fund	Introduction of a new maximum age for entering health insurance schemes and coverage for the self-employed	1996, 1997

Sources: ISSA, Data Base "Developments and Trends"; Aidi Hu, "China: Innovations in health care financing—Mixing individual and collective responsibility," in ISSR, 3/97, pp. 51-74.

Funding Adjustments

Several of the countries in this region have found it necessary to make adjustments to funding, particularly with regard to the level of contributions and increases therein.

In India the contribution assessment ceiling has been raised to such an extent that approximately one million further employees can be made statutorily liable to pay contributions. Employees thus pay 1.75 percent of salary as contribution, while employers pay 4.75 percent. This is offset by increases in daily sickness allowances.

In Korea efforts are under way, as part of the current reform, to bring all the existing insurance funds together into a single fund. By unifying all the associated risk the government hopes to achieve not only a single area of financial compensation, but also improvements in equality of access to health care and efficiency.[11]

The Chinese health care system also hopes to achieve such aims with the new directions it is adopting, combining elements from the approach for social insurance schemes with those of provident funds.[12]

Plans are in hand in Japan for a comprehensive reorganization of financial regulations comprising not only increases in contributions by employers and employees but also additional personal contributions and cost sharing payments. These arrangements cover such things as the 10 percent increase in payments for prescription drugs, the prescription fee and cost sharing payments for hospital visits going up to JPY 2,000 per month.

Including the Poor in Social Protection in the Case of Sickness

In India the introduction of a new health insurance scheme resulted in the inclusion of over four million people under coverage for hospital treatment in the first year receiving cost reimbursements of up to INR.5,000 per year. This new insurance scheme is intended exclusively for the poor and is financed solely from contributions. The scheme is intended to cover the agricultural population and industrial workers. Table 1.7 above provides details.

Measures have also been introduced to provide coverage for the informal sector in the Indian population.[13]

Table 1.7
India: Introduction of a New Health Insurance Scheme for the Poor and
Contribution Increases for Employers and Employees

The Government of India has introduced a new health insurance scheme for the poor. In its first year this scheme, Janarogya Yojana, will cover over four million persons between the ages of 5 and 70. It is a social, non-profit-making scheme.

Comprehensive health insurance coverage is being offered by four insurance companies. Insurance coverage is up to INR5,000 per year covering hospitalisation for up to 30 days, and 60 days after release from hospital.

Contributions will be low so that the poor in agricultural areas and industrial workers in the cities can join the scheme.

In the context of the State insurance scheme for employees, the contribution assessment level has been raised from INR 3,000 to INR 6,500 to include approximately another million employees. Contribution rates have been raised from 4 percent to 4.75 percent of employer payroll figures. In return benefits have been extended. The daily cash sickness allowance has been raised from INR 53 to INRR 125.

Reference: Ministry of Labour Notification, 23 December 1996.

Sources: International Federation of Health Funds, *FHF Newsletter*, January 1997; Employees' State Insurance Corporation, ISSA Data Base "Developments and Trends."

Europe: Benefit Adjustments with Regard to Demographic Trends and Introduction of Market Forces in Health Care Schemes

Health care systems in Europe over the past three years have been characterized by the introduction of new benefits and the implementation of fundamental reforms.[14] The aims of the measures adopted here are to

- control rising costs occasioned by long-term population ageing[15];

- redistribute roles between the state and market forces; and

- introduce new information technologies.

Table 1.8 presents an overview of the most important reforms. The reforms in Luxemburg and the Netherlands are presented in more detail.

Table 1.8
Selected Reforms in Social Protection in the Case of Sickness in Europe,
1996-1998, by Country

Country	Health care system	Reform	Date of implementation
Germany	Social insurance scheme	Introduction of a long-term care insurance scheme	1995, 1996
		Increased co-payments, introduction of free choice of insurance scheme, admission of contribution reimbursement and franchise, introduction of a flat charge for hospital financing	1997
France	Social insurance scheme	Restructuring of social security and cost containment	2000
		Introduction of long-term care allowances	1997
Greece	Social insurance scheme	Restructuring of the national health service	??
Israel	Social insurance scheme	Abolition of parallel tax to ease the burden on employers	1997
Latvia	Social insurance scheme Universal health care system	Introduction of social tax contributions	1996
Lithuania	Social insurance scheme Universal health care system	Introduction of a health insurance system	1997
Luxemburg	Social insurance system	Introduction of a long-term care insurance scheme	1998
Netherlands	Social insurance scheme	Privatization of health insurance for employees	1996
Austria	Social insurance scheme	Cuts of long-term case benefits. Revision of hospital financing	1997
Switzerland	Social insurance scheme	Revision of health insurance and cost containment	1996, 1997
Spain	Social insurance scheme	Free choice of physician for specialist treatment	1996
Hungary	Social insurance scheme	Reduction in cash sickness allowance	1996

Source: ISSA Data Base "Developments and Trends."

Taking Account of Long-Term Population Trends

The reforms in Germany, Luxemburg, and France, and to some extent Austria, address population ageing and the concomitant increase in the requirement for long-term care in each health insurance system.

The insurance scheme for long-term care in Germany grants benefits for both care in the home and in institutions. The benefits for care in the home are organized in a standard three-tier system and can take the form of either money payments or benefits in kind. Hospital, or nursing home care, is paid for up to a maximum amount. The insurance scheme is financed from contributions. A non-working public holiday was abolished to compensate employers for the additional contribution burden. The Länder meet investment costs for nursing homes, etc.

Table 1.9
Luxemburg: Introduction of a Long-Term Care Insurance Scheme

A Bill introducing a scheme, largely based on the German model, was put before the Chamber of Deputies and has now been adopted. Its main principles are:

- An emphasis on maintaining people at home, rather than on caring for them in an institution;
- An emphasis on benefits in kind, rather than on benefits in cash;
- The establishment of three degrees of dependency;
- The adaptation of the benefit according to the degree of dependency, with the possibility of combining benefits in kind with cash benefits;
- Adequate social protection for family members who provide care;
- Mixed financing consisting of contributions based on taxable income and a contribution from the State budget.

At the beginning of 1998, the Bill concerning the introduction of a dependency insurance scheme in Luxemburg was still pending with the competent parliamentary authorities. Proposed amendments contained provision, in particular, for the notion of costs payable according to individual need instead of according to the degree of dependency.

Reference: Ministère de la Sécurité sociale, Projet de loi portant introduction d'une assurance dépendance.

Sources: Association luxembourgeoise des organismes de sécurité sociale, ISSA Data Base "Developments and Trends."

As table 1.9 sets out in more detail, the reform Bill that was introduced was similar to the one introduced in Germany in 1995-1996 and contains provisions for dependency insurance, benefits in kind, and to a certain extent, also cash benefits. Unlike the German legislation, however, the extent of benefits is not calculated according to a standard degree of dependency, but is to be determined according to each individual case.

Some time ago, France introduced benefits for aged dependents in one test area. These benefits, which are now to be introduced on a countrywide basis, replace the existing compensation of dependents through benefits in kind, which are determined by degree of dependency.

Austria has been obliged to cut back benefits in view of the high cost of care. This has involved a reduction in the attendance allowance. Hospital financing has also had to be redesigned in order to put a stop to cost-driven inflation.

The efforts to take into account population trends in Europe also contain a greater focus on benefits in the areas of prevention and rehabilitation.[16]

Responsibility Sharing between the Market and the State

Other countries are attempting to cope with rising costs by a deeper involvement of market elements in health care provision, or by schemes largely organized by the private sector.

Thus, the Netherlands has abolished most statutory cash sickness benefits, since these benefits have been "privatized," that is to say they are no longer paid by the state social security system but by the employer. This is expected to lead to annual savings of NLG 900 million of taxpayers' money, and also to help combat absenteeism. Table 1.10 provides further details.

Similarly, measures have also been taken in Switzerland. A new law has introduced a basic compulsory insurance scheme and a complementary insurance scheme, for which private insurance companies are largely responsible. Insured persons are free to choose their insurance company and to change insurers to encourage competitiveness. However, the list of benefits under the basic insurance scheme is laid down by law.

In the interests of cost containment, Germany is also counting on the introduction of private insurance elements. Thus, henceforth,

Table 1.10
Netherlands: Privatization of Social Health Insurance for Employees

As a result of the Act on the extension of the obligation for employers to continue wage payments in case of sickness (WULBZ), the Dutch health insurance scheme for insured persons engaged in regular employment has been "privatized." Most of the compulsory sickness benefits under the Sickness Benefits Act (ZW) will no longer be payable. Instead, employers are now required to pay 70 percent of a sick worker's wages for a period of 52 weeks. Daily sickness allowances previously paid out of a collective fund to salaried employees of private enterprises were abolished with effect from 1 March 1996.

The health insurance financed out of collective social funds has been maintained as a safety net for certain categories of persons, who are unemployed, or no longer employed. It also covers employees in need of special protection, such as employees who are basically entitled to continued wage payments in whose case, however, the legislator is of the opinion that the burden on the employer in respect of this payment obligation would not be advisable. Workers on maternity leave, disabled workers resuming work, and workers in special employment relationships—such as home workers and some stand-by workers—are examples of persons who continue to be entitled to sickness benefits out of collective social funds.

Obligation for employers to continue wage payments in case of sickness
For other categories of people, the employer is obliged to pay employees on sick leave 70 percent of their wage or salary, up to a ceiling set in 1996 at NLG 75,583. The WULBZ contains safeguards against employers attempting to circumvent their obligations by adjusting the employment contract. On the other hand, the WULBZ stipulates that entitlement to continued wage payment during the first day, or the first two days, of sick leave can be excluded through collective agreements. Employers will have the option of taking out full or partial insurance against the financial risk of their employees' sickness.

Combatting absenteeism and tax savings
The Government expects this measure to result in annual savings of NLG 900 million for the State and to help in combatting absenteeism. Under the terms of the Working Conditions Act (Arbowet) employers are required to call in what is known as an "Arbodienst" (a private certified working conditions consultancy) to monitor absence through sick leave and supervise sick workers. The purpose of these activities is to ensure that employees resume (suitable) work as soon as possible. The employer has the right to require full co-operation of an employee in occupational rehabilitation programs. Non-compliance can be sanctioned by loss of entitlement to continued wage payments; in the case of refusal to co-operate the worker also loses entitlement to sickness benefits from collective funds.

Implications for contribution payments
Enactment of WULBZ also implied the abolition of ZW contribution payments, which were as follows: insured person: 10.95 percent of earnings; employer: 8.2 percent of payroll, including 7.25 percent for medical benefits and 0.95 percent for cash benefits; Government: cost of supplements necessary to top up cash sickness benefits to a guaranteed minimum income level. To finance the remaining ZW benefits, i.e., those paid to the special groups of persons listed above, contributions to the unemployment benefit scheme are to be increased.

Source: ISSA Data Base "Developments and Trends."

the compulsory health insurance system allows the possibility of contributions reimbursement and franchise. Furthermore, insured persons' freedom to choose their own insurance scheme has been introduced in Germany.

A radical restructuring of health care has also been carried out in France in the context of the revision of the social welfare system. The reform is intended to contain the increasing social welfare deficits, in particular, through a redefinition of competencies for the State and for administrative bodies, new regulatory mechanisms for outpatient treatment, and the re-organization of hospital management and financing.

The Use of New Information Technologies

The use of new information technologies in the further development of health care systems is largely aimed at improving efficiency.[17]

Achievements hoped for are a more rational organization of tasks, the substitution of electronic records for paper records, the removal of sources of errors and unnecessary repetitions.

Aims also include a qualitative improvement in treatment through case and disease management, guidelines and hospital monitoring. Further areas where new technologies are expected to be introduced are needs analysis and finance allocation. The use of new technologies, however, also touches on problems of data protection.[18]

Summarizing, it can be stated that the reforms in many developing countries are often directed at extending coverage to include more population groups and at restructuring health care systems. In industrialized countries attempts are being made to strike a more contemporary balance between the economics of the market and social policy demands, as well as deal with needs of ageing populations.

What is clear is that developments and trends over recent years have been focusing on improving the equity in access to health care, while at the same time trying to overcome financial shortfalls through cost control. These efforts are supported by measures to optimize institutional frameworks, improve benefit quality and to help health care systems move forward through the introduction of new information technologies.

The contributions that follow in this publication present the innovative solutions found for these areas in detail and how these solutions are to be evaluated. However, the reader should not expect global models for social health insurance, but rather experiences concerning the best practices, successes, and failures which can support sound development in each individual country.

Notes

1. Cf. Schieber, G. Maeda, A. 1997."A Curmudgeon's guide to financing health care in developing countries," in World Bank, An International Conference, "Innovations in health care financing," Washington D.C., March 10-11.
2. Cf. here Maynard, A. 1998. "Making difficult choices in health care," in *Summit of international managed care trends*, Delegate Handbook, Informational Resource Kit, December 9-12, Miami Beach.
3. Cf. here details from the contribution by Duranton, M., Zuaq, A., Pilón, P. in this publication.
4. Cf. Chollet, D. et al. 1997. "Private Insurance: Principles and Practice," in *Innovations in Health Care Financing*, World Bank, Washington.
5. Cf. de Wet, E. 1997. "Reformtendenzen im südafrikanischen Gesundheits- und Krankenversicherungs-system: eine erste Bilanz," in *Zeitschrift für Sozialreform*, 87, S. 477-492.
6. Cf. here contribution by Ron, A. and van Ginneken, W. in this publication with examples from numerous developing countries.
7. Cf. here for details of the contribution by Duranton, M., Zuaq,A., and Pilón, J. in this publication.
8. Cf. Krause, J. 1997. *Das Krankenversicherungssystem der USA*, Baden-Baden, p.125 ff.
9. Cf. contribution by Newbrander, W. and Eichler, R. in this publication.
10. Cf. here for details of the contribution by Iguchi, N. in this publication.
11. Cf. here National Health Insurance Corporation, National Health Insurance in the Republic of Korea, Seoul, 1999.
12. Cf. here the contribution by Hu, A. in this publication.
13. Cf. here the contribution by van Ginneken, W. in this publication.
14. Cf. here the contribution by Duranton , M., Zuaq, A., and Pilon, P. in this publication.
15. Benefit direction with regard to population ageing is not only confined to Europe but also applies to Japan. Cf. here the contributions by Iguchi N. and Scheil-Adlung, X. in this publication.
16. Cf. here the contributions by Müller-Fahrnow, W. in this publication.
17. Cf. here the contributions by Delaveau, C. and Brenner, G. in this publication.
18. Cf. here the Contribution by Blobel, B. in this publication.

Part 2

New Approaches in Extending Health Care Coverage

2

New Strategies for the Formal Sector: Focus on Vietnam and Zimbabwe

A. Ron

The focus of this publication is on recent innovations in social health insurance. The review of extension of coverage concentrates on developing countries. With the exception of very few developing countries, the introduction of both short-term and long-term social security benefits lagged behind in the period of rapid economic development in the 1970s and 1980s.

After several decades of steady, sometimes very rapid economic development, we have more recently had situations ranging from slow growth, through recession and economic crisis as well as through transition from planned to market economies. In some countries and spanning the same time period, long periods of civil unrest followed independence from colonial rule. A review of the extension of health insurance should be considered within this background. The formal sector population is dealt with first, followed by a separate chapter on the informal sector. For the purposes of this publication, the term formal sector covers active and retired workers, as well as their dependents, in both public and private labor sectors. The term workers includes salaried and self-employed individuals, in permanent, temporary, or seasonal employment. In addition to nationals working in the country, migrant and overseas worker categories should be included. In this context, we would define the formal sector as covering workers in registered commercial and non-commercial enterprises, with continuation of their status or affiliation through periods of invalidity and retirement.

During periods of civil unrest and economic crises, organized labor pressures tends to be suppressed, particularly in the private sector. In some countries with a large civil service, a relatively generous range of health and welfare benefits were provided to these
workers and their dependents. Although these services were generally insufficient compensation for low public sector salaries, the free
care nature of these benefits may well have reduced pressure for a
contributory social health insurance mechanism from public sector
workers.

When some stability is achieved, aggressive investment policies
may take precedence over issues related to workers rights, including safe working conditions. Both multinational and national investors, particularly those willing to establish manufacturing enterprises
for export, were given a range of tax exemption privileges. In some
countries, the exemptions extended to existing social security
schemes and even work safety regulations were ignored. This happened in many countries, and perhaps the example of Bangladesh is
most pertinent. Reviews of working conditions and health of the
garment workers in Bangladesh (Islam, 1997) illustrate both the need
for social health insurance and the complexities of establishing viable schemes. Garment workers now comprise over 4 million workers, 90 percent are young women, with an average age of 19.5 years,
and they are likely to stay in the industry for three to four years.
Worker turnover is high, and many women change jobs several times
a year, as better wages and better conditions are found. Most are
migrant workers, coming from districts far from the factories. Some
live in hostels while most live in makeshift urban slum dwellings
within a 5-mile radius from their jobs. Their earnings were calculated to be 35 percent below minimum wage in Bangladesh if over-
time pay was not included.

The garment factory conditions were characterized by poor ventilation, inadequate lighting, no seating at the workbench, restricted
use of inadequate drinking water, unhygienic sanitation facilities and
no canteen for meal breaks. Compensation for work-related injuries
and accidents were limited, following a Labour Law of 1923 which
covers only permanent workers. Most factories in this fairly new
industry have been set up in rented houses which are inappropriate
for such production activities. The enormous potential labor force,
limited job opportunities and the lack of government funds and in-

spection capacity for factory safety and hygiene all combined to suppress demands for basic working conditions and social protection. Some pressure has only recently been generated by international aid agencies, following factory fires resulting in a high number of fatalities.

Another factor that has affected the extension of social health insurance coverage is globalization. Trade liberalization as well as modern communications have led to increased movement of labor between countries. The traditional protection mechanisms developed for seamen have not been carried in to the current large scale labor migrations. Social protection, including health insurance is provided for a very small proportion of migrant workers today. Most migrant workers go from countries with low social security coverage, and have not considered social protection, including their health care, as a factor in the attractiveness of the job market in the country in which they found jobs. Any perceived lack of social protection has been only one of the disadvantages faced by migrant workers (Weinert, 1991, Bohning, 1996). On the side of the receiving countries with well-developed health insurance coverage, many non-national workers, particularly those coming from developing countries to domestic employment, may not have benefited from the national regulations.

In parallel, we are now witnessing a decrease in interest among young workers in social security in the host industrialized countries. At all levels of education, from high school dropouts to university graduates, the young workers entering the job market may be willing to forego both job security through tenure and social protection for the opportunity to be employed at all or for job advancement.

For also these reasons, only a minority of workers, and mainly those in the public and private salaried labor sectors of developing countries, benefit from any form of income replacement in old age and from access to health care through social insurance mechanisms. National schemes developed for these contingencies seemed to work quite well, but very little attention was paid to low coverage and to compliance with both the registration of workers and collection of contributions. In the new schemes developed in several Asian countries in the early 1990s, such as Thailand, and Vietnam, compulsory health insurance coverage was established for workers only, rather than for the wage-earner and dependents. The administrative complexity and lack of information on expected utilization and costs of benefits deterred the new systems from taking on dependents. Many schemes claimed that during their evolutionary stage, they simply did not have the administrative capacity to extend coverage to such categories as workers in enterprises with less than 10 or even 20 employees, to workers within family businesses, domestic workers or to the self-employed. Since such workers were generally not members of any organized labor associations, and tended not be involved in any other form of solidarity groups, there was little pressure to extend health insurance coverage to these individuals (Atim, 1994).

If we look at the situation today, we are likely to find that the volume of this previously insured population has not grown and may even have shrunk in volume. The historical events mentioned above, such as independence followed by civil unrest, economic transition or crisis, were the more obvious reasons for a decrease in coverage as a proportion of the total population. In parallel, there were the latent pressures to avoid the extension of social security to salaried workers, such as the efforts to maintain preferential low labor costs in the competitive and increasingly global market. Most of the existing coverage was through broad social security schemes, which lacked the administrative capacity to take on new groups. Some past lack of understanding of social health insurance within the health sector probably contributed to the stagnation of the extent of coverage. In the interim, the majority of the population had access to basic but limited health services, including both preventive and curative care, in public facilities, while the minority increasingly purchased care from the growing availability of private health care providers.

In the past there was a general lack of awareness and interest in extending both benefits and coverage, and the complacency of all the stakeholders did not promote serious action to improve the systems. Several factors have begun to shake us out of this complacency resulting in vigorous new initiatives to extend coverage from several sources. First is the pressure to decrease public expenditure, with across the board implications for government activities. Several countries have embarked on streamlining their civil service and reducing fringe benefits for staff and their dependents. This includes shifting to contributory prepayment mechanisms for health care which may then be merged into the existing social insurance systems for the private sector. Such a shift is indeed necessary for the economic reforms which focus on privatization of state enterprises.

At the same time, the dramatic reduction in public funds for health care placed the emphasis on health care as the priority benefit in social security development, involving a new set of agencies outside of the traditional tripartite partners: ministries of labor and social welfare, employers and workers associations. This led to new initiatives from ministries of health, following changes in health care financing policies. Within the health system reforms now taking place, many countries faced with public expenditure reduction view health insurance as the optimal mechanism to finance health care. When these ministries of health are also the major health care providers in the country, the growth of health insurance coverage is also necessary to ensure revenues for their already existing but increasingly under-funded facilities. The recognized negative impact of imposing user charges in public hospitals before social safety nets are in place is now increasing the pressures for universal health insurance (Abel-Smith, 1992). The decisions on the new health care financing options also need to take into account changes in demography and morbidity patterns. Life expectancy has increased in most countries, more people will live longer, with more chronic diseases to be detected and treated for longer periods, and the costs of health care increase at a pace faster than those of any other goods and services, for a variety of reasons.

A third and related factor follows analysis of the impact of economic crises, including the recent events in Asia (Robb and Zhang, 1988). The negative social impact of regional and national economic crises have increased recognition of the role of social safety nets, including social protection in the form of health insurance, directly on health and access to health care and in avoiding poverty.

Recent Innovations

To illustrate what has been done recently to extend social health insurance coverage in the formal sector, experiences in two countries, Vietnam and Zimbabwe, are described. They are of course, vastly different, not only in geographical location, but also in the context of the development of social health insurance. In Vietnam, the experience described is part of the development of a national health insurance scheme, covering various population sectors in stages, through both compulsory and voluntary components, until universal coverage is reached. Health insurance development is part of a health system reform process, following government policies in all areas of social and economic transition. The introduction of health insurance signifies the adoption of social insurance as the optimal mechanism to finance health care within this process.

In Zimbabwe, national policies regarding health care financing have not yet been finalized, despite at least a decade of recognition of the inability of the government to provide adequate funding for health care. The relatively large-scale development of social health insurance followed non-government initiatives, driven by employer concerns for workers' welfare, recognition of the advantages of pooling risks and funds beyond the enterprise level, as well the advantages of the administration of recognized workers' benefits by agencies outside their own enterprise management.

Vietnam

Background. The introduction of health insurance in Vietnam is relatively recent, beginning with the national Vietnam Health Insurance Decree in August 1992. (Carrin and Ron, 1998) Since 1987, the economic and political climate changed rapidly with the move from a centrally planned to a market-based economy. An integral part of this reform was the fiscal policy calling for a reduction in public expenditure, including cuts in allocations for health care. As a result, the health sector was under pressure to find alternatives to public resources for health, previously generated from central to provincial and district levels.

The government recognized the need for cost-sharing with the population, and accepted health insurance as the viable option to finance health care. In August 1992 the government issued the first national Health Insurance Decree, with both compulsory and voluntary health insurance components. This decree was immediately followed by the implementation of health insurance in several provinces, based on the limited experience of pilot schemes in several provinces (Carrin et al., 1993). Overall responsibility for policy development was placed with the Department of Finance and Planning of the Ministry of Health. Implementation was carried out through the Vietnam Health Insurance (VHI) which was established as the a separate authority within the Ministry of Health to implement both compulsory and voluntary health insurance throughout the country. The VHI operates as a state company within the Ministry of Health, under a Vice Minister for Health charged with this responsibility. Supervision is statutorily the responsibility of a Health Insurance Board, chaired by another Vice Minister of Health and with members from within the Ministry of Health and other ministries. Administration of the scheme is decentralized to provincial VHI offices, which have relative flexibility in determining contribution rates for voluntary insurance and contractual arrangements with providers.

The Health Insurance Decree of 1992 stipulated coverage of all salaried and retired workers in the public sector and all salaried workers in the private sector. The decree gave eligibility for benefits to the workers only, and dependents of the insured could enroll in the voluntary insurance channel, which was primarily designed for the rural farmer population and the self-employed. There were basically five categories of insured persons under both compulsory and voluntary insurance: active and retired government administrative workers, industrial workers, agricultural workers and other self-employed, spouses and other adult citizens, and children between 6 and 16 years old.

The target population for health insurance coverage currently does not include military and police personnel, and children under 6 years of age. Individuals in these population groups are by law entitled to care free of charge in public health facilities. Also excluded were residents of Mountain Area villages, most of which are in areas now termed "New Economic Areas," with special taxation and economic development benefits.

In many provinces, schoolchildren (over the age of 6 years) were insured under a general insurance policy developed by the Viet Insurance Company (Bao Viet), which is the state company dealing with liability insurance for property, motor vehicles, and other general areas. This situation meant that three parallel health insurance schemes were in operation from 1993, and that different members of the same family could be in one of the three schemes, with different contribution levels and different benefits. In addition, several state enterprises, such as coal mining, rubber, oil and gas companies, initially set up their own insurance schemes. No standard methods to cover very low-income or non-economically active individuals were promulgated during that period, but provinces were encouraged to introduce forms of support, particularly for poor populations, through local government, national, and international agencies.

By 1994 it was reported that close to 4.5 million persons or 5.5 percent of the total population were insured: 2.5 million salaried workers, 1.5 million retired civil servants and the rest under voluntary insurance in the 53 provinces. These figures implied that close to 90 percent of public sector active salaried workers and over 90 percent of public sector retirees were registered. Government ministries transferred the contributions for their employees as well as retirees on a regular basis. However, many small state enterprises claimed that they were unable to pay the contributions (set at 3 percent of salary, with 2 percent paid by employer and 1 percent by the worker), creating a discrepancy between registration and actual continued coverage.

At that stage, it was realized that major efforts would be required to extend coverage, and strategies to do so were developed for specific target populations. Besides the overall goal of reaching universal coverage, the composition of the insured population in itself posed serious financial risks. One-third of the 4.5 million persons covered in 1995 were retired civil servants, with the corresponding morbidity of their age group, while the membership had very few private sector workers, with high contribution amounts but low risks.

Strategies were developed to extend coverage, through both the compulsory and voluntary components to four specific target groups: Family members of the compulsory insured, the very low-income population, schoolchildren and students in higher education, and salaried workers in the private and public sector.

Family members of workers covered by compulsory insurance. For the first category, attempts were made in several provinces to first strengthen compliance in the population covered by compulsory insurance, and thereby to broaden the extension of coverage. Insured workers were offered a significantly discounted rate to enroll their dependents, as long as all members of the family were covered in order to minimize adverse selection. Employers were encouraged but not compelled to share part of the family member contribution. When first introduced in selected provinces in 1995, the option was not taken up by the expected number of workers, as indeed there were few incentives for the individual or household to voluntarily pay for health insurance. At that time, there was deterioration rather than improvement in conditions in hospitals and commune health services. The introduction of user charges, which indeed was part of the policy towards cost-recovery and the introduction of health insurance as the option, failed to generate incentives to purchase the health cards. Initially, the user charges were low and even below real costs for some services.

Under the first health insurance decree there was also some lack of clarification regarding the benefits covered particularly in ambulatory care. The comprehensive nature of the benefits was clarified in 1995 through circulars related to the decree, while the decree itself was amended in January 1998.

An additional problem was administrative capacity of the scheme at provincial and district levels. The new provincial VHI offices and district branches could only manage annual contribution collection. While the monthly contribution was considered affordable for the majority of the population, the amounts needed to cover one year's membership was not acceptable. While the concept of the family discount was clear, all the proposals had to be approved by the provincial VHI board, and this process was lengthy and complex for a new institution.

Several lessons were learnt from these attempts, mainly in Ninh Binh province. The first was that voluntary health insurance is not attractive when benefits are not clear. A second was that annual registration and contribution is not compatible with the marketing of voluntary insurance. Both issues were addressed by 1998 and the same approach of the family package was then successfully launched in the population covered by the Rubber Company of Vietnam. This state enterprise is responsible for the health insurance coverage of its workers in eight provinces, operating as a VHI provincial office. In this case, the company could develop its own proposals regarding the contribution level and pledged to share the contribution with the workers. The family membership option was launched in 1998 for the 750,000 population covered.

Very low-income population. The efforts to cover the very low-income families were started in Hai Phong province, which focused on covering individuals and family members recognized as recipients of welfare allowances through local government funds. The provincial government, through the People's Committee, purchased annual health insurance membership cards for distribution to the recognized list of welfare recipients. In 1998, over 200,000 cards were provided to this target population. The granting of free cards to this population significantly increased coverage at the provincial level to 42 percent of the total population in that year. The method was later used to purchase cards for welfare recipients in Hanoi and Nghe An provinces. While the individuals covered are not formal sector workers, this social assistance mechanism in fact constitutes a mechanism to extend coverage through a "free card" system for the indigent population, through the existing social insurance system. The method is also important in the promotion of equity and removal of discriminatory features in providing health care to the disadvantaged population as the cards are identical to those in other categories of insured persons.

The attention to the low income families was quite unrelated to coverage of the social group population. This group now comprises around one million of the 10 million covered by VHI by mid-1999 and includes persons with meritorious services to the revolution, invalids, orphans of veterans, and heroes' mothers. The coverage is mandated by a government ordinance issued at the end of 1995 regarding special social support for such individuals. The Ministry of Labour, Invalids and Social Affairs (MOLISA) directly pays VHI the flat-rate premiums for these individuals.

Schoolchildren. The third target group for the extension of coverage was schoolchildren aged 6 years and over and students in higher education. The initiative to concentrate on this group resulted partly from an effort to shift the health component from the school insurance policies offered by the State Viet Insurance Company to the VHI. From 1995/96 school year, about half of the VHI provincial offices had initiated school health insurance, with Hai Phong covering 80 percent of the target population and Ho Chi Minh City covering 45 percent in 1998.

In the first stage, fixed percentages of the revenues were allocated to health provided in the schools, inpatient care, incentives to the teachers for registration and contribution collection and administration of the scheme. In Ho Chi Minh City, 10 percent of the revenues were allocated to cover children whose parents could not afford the flat-rate contribution, which was set at increasing levels according to school level. Over time, it became clear that these allocations did not correspond to needs. The 45 percent allocation for services in the schools led to waste, particularly in the form of drugs purchased for the school clinic, while the inpatient allocation led to unnecessary hospitalization of schoolchildren. By 1998, when over 3 million children were covered, changes were made in the allocations and the hospital-based benefits were increased to cover more outpatient services, based on a study of some 2,000 children in primary schools in Ho Chi Minh province (VHI, 1998). The allocations for school services were changed substantially to include preventive services, such as safe drinking water and sanitation, as well as health education.

Two very positive outcomes of the coverage of schoolchildren should be noted. First was the cooperation that developed between the various government agencies responsible for the health of children, and the VHI. The Ministry of Education and Training is statutorily responsible for school health. Through the development of the program for the coverage of schoolchildren, the VHI facilitated continued collaboration between the Ministry of Health, Ministry of Education and Training as well as the VHI itself at national and provincial levels. One result was the development of school health programs to meet current needs at the local level. The second outcome was the awareness of social health insurance introduced to the families through the coverage of their children. For many families, particularly those in which the parents are self-employed, this was their first encounter with the concepts of prepayment for defined health care benefits.

Salaried workers. The fourth target was the active salaried worker population, with emphasis on the private sector. The increase in the number of insured persons in this sector was minimal over the first five years of VHI operation. During this period there was slow privatization of state enterprises, with many of their workers as well as young university graduates starting small businesses. Many joint ventures were also set up during this period, mainly in the southern provinces of Vietnam. Inadequate registration of private enterprises was initially a serious problem, while those registered tended not to report all the workers on their payroll or under-reported their salaries. Typically, review of the contribution revenues from many individual enterprises showed that the calculation base was the minimum wage for the occupational sector, or a contract salary which is far below actual earnings. The use of this calculation base may be linked to old practices in centrally planned economies, where standard salaries were common.

Compliance with the registration of new workers covered by compulsory insurance has improved only marginally with better registration of enterprises. In 1997, the VHI conducted interviews of employers and workers in private enterprises registered in selected areas of Hanoi (VHI 1998) failed to find around half of the 558 the small business included in the lists, which came from municipal licensing sources. Among the 106 enterprises (with over 10 workers) surveyed, only 13 percent had registered their workers, while 15 percent of the 1,200 workers interviewed replied that they had valid VHI membership cards. These findings are very similar to the reported extent of registration in pension schemes, administered by the Ministry of Labour, Invalids and Social Affairs.

One of the major reasons for the failure to register workers in the private sector was highlighted by this survey. As with the voluntary insurance described above, contribution was done on a prepayment basis, usually for 6 months, following which new cards were printed and issued for validity for the period of this prepayment. Private sector enterprises could not meet the cash outlay which this method required, particularly as their revenues were dependent on a new market environment. The findings promoted changes, and led the VHI to change to a monthly contribution collection system in early in 1999. The change requires far more than the actual updating of enterprises and workers along with the transfer of funds. The VHI has had to change the system of producing and issuing cards to a longer-term system, in which the validity of the card is linked to payments made for the past rather than future period.

From the information available on compliance, it is not clear to what extent this means that higher paid workers are still left out. Labor statistics indicate that the major joint ventures, with large numbers of workers and higher wages, have not registered their regular workers. Very few of these enterprises, particularly those in manufacturing companies, were listed in the Hanoi and Ho Chi Minh provincial VHI offices at the time. The situation was far worse in other provinces. In Nghe An for example, the Labour Union reported 43,000 workers in private enterprises in 1997. At that time, only one company had registered its 100 workers and was contributing to VHI in the entire province.

There has been considerable improvement in the reporting of wages since implementation of an agreement with the income tax authorities (at provincial level) in 1995, whereby information on real wages paid is relayed to the VHI. The Ministry of Finance, which is responsible for income tax assessment and collection, introduced regulations allowing for the blocking of an enterprise bank account in such cases of non-compliance with social insurance regulations. In the last year, differences in the calculated versus actual contribution paid (on the basis of wages reported) were collected from the enterprises and passed on to the insurance. As compliance is increased, particularly regarding the reporting of wages, it will be necessary to introduce relevant ceilings. At present, the 3 percent contribution is deducted on the reported salary.

However, basic constraints with the extension of coverage for this group remain in the nature of the Health Insurance Decree, including the amended Decree of 1998. As a decree rather than law, sanctions against employers who do not register their workers are very limited. Linkage with income tax authorities may not be the optimal solution, particularly in developing countries where the establishment of broad and fair taxation systems represents a problem in itself. While the health sector reform policy clearly looks towards universal health insurance as the mechanism to finance health care, steps to draft legislation (rather than a decree), with the appropriate sanctions for non-compliance, have not yet been taken. In addition, the most rapid growth in private enterprise has been in small businesses with less than 10 workers, which is the starting number of workers for compulsory coverage. Small enterprises with less than 10 workers comprised close to 60 percent those listed and found in the study conducted by the VHI in 1997, as noted above. There is also a need to examine a trend to engage workers on temporary or piece-work bases, in order to avoid payment of employer contributions to health insurance as well as other levies.

Summary of the extension of coverage in Vietnam. To summarize the problems related to the extension of coverage for this group, compliance is the major issue, impeded by the lack of awareness and sanctions. Motivation on the part of the workers is low when only the worker is covered while family members are more likely to need care. The situation has recently been compounded by the introduction of a co-payment of 20 percent of the charges for health care, to be made by the patient at the time of use. The decision to introduce the co-payment was made to deal with abuse of the system, although the sources of abuse are mainly on the provider side, in the form of extremely high use of prescribed drugs and ancillary diagnostic services in both outpatient and inpatient care. The VHI itself did not initiate co-payments, as there is good understanding of the implications for motivation for any population group to join the scheme under such conditions. Since 1995, user charges in public facilities have increased at least fivefold, and a co-payment of 20 percent could be a serious deterrent to seeking care. A single admission for minor surgery could result in a co-payment by the patient amounting to twice the average monthly earnings.

It is also accepted that the irrational utilization patterns which characterize the abuse stem from provider rather than patient behavior. The continued use of the fee-for-service provider payment system has led to more rather than less abuse. As health insurance accounts for an increasing proportion of the provider revenues, the ability to generate even more revenues is realized and aggressively applied. Since the health care delivery system is a public system, operated by the Ministry of Health at central and decentralized levels, there have been attempts to curb such abuse through Ministerial circulars. Efforts are also made through the re-negotiation of contracts between the provincial VHI offices and the public providers serving their insured populations. There is increasing interest in the VHI to introduce capitation provider payment systems, and to control abuse without patient co-payments.

In describing the membership situation at present, several features of the health insurance system in Vietnam should be noted. First, the compulsory scheme covers active and retired workers, and not their dependents. Second, the compulsory scheme has included retired public sector workers since its inception, which imposed a burden on a new scheme, as utilization and expenditure for the elderly are more than twice the average for the total insured population. The fund also does not have the benefit of reserves from past contributions from the retired workers during their years of economic activity, as in the case of established schemes. In the first two years of implementation, the retired constituted more than 50 percent of the insured population. They now constitute 30 percent and this proportion will obviously decline over time, but the proportion will remain high compared to other national social health insurance systems.

Contributions of the salaried workers therefore heavily subsidize retired workers rather than dependents of the same worker. The lack of benefits for the worker's family members also diminishes interest in health insurance. The workers themselves may have considerably less need than their children. The current approach to having dependents enrolled through a voluntary mechanism may also have negative implications regarding equity. Workers with lower salary levels or workers in low-income enterprises may be less prepared to enroll their dependents. So far the contributions for dependents is the same flat-rate amount, regardless of the individual worker's salary. As the salaried sector grows in Vietnam, it would obviously be faster and fairer to extend coverage if dependents were automatically covered through the compulsory insurance mechanism, through an adjusted contribution based on percentage of salary.

Another issue in considering the extension of membership towards universal coverage is the current provision regarding children. A decree of 1995 stipulated that health care for children under 6 years is free, that is, financed by the MOH through general revenues. In practice, the level of funding is determined mainly by provincial level resources. As government funding is basically low (reported to be US$3.00 per person in 1994), reliance on public funds for the health care of children does not necessarily imply an adequate level of funding in all provinces. Here again, the inclusion of children as dependents rather than in a separate category needs to be reconsidered. The inclusion of all children would also facilitate the conventional family approach to health insurance, whereby all family members could be covered through compulsory insurance for the salaried workers. The target population for voluntary insurance would then be the self-employed sector, at least until compulsory universal coverage can be implemented.

The government of Vietnam decided in mid-1999 to provide an annual allocation to purchase health insurance cards for the poor. Initial estimates were that up to 10 million individuals would be covered through this allocation. While this is a very positive development, parallel efforts will be needed to increase coverage in other population sectors. It would be unfortunate if the considerable efforts of the VHI are undermined by the perception of this national scheme as a health insurance fund for low-income populations. The extension of coverage through better compliance in the private salaried worker sector is therefore important, as this remains the only option for strengthening the financial viability of the fund, and retaining the advantages of the broad opportunities for pooling in the original design of social health insurance in Vietnam.

Payment for health services provided to the insured in government health care facilities accounted to around 20 percent of the Ministry of Health budget by mid-1996. However, in some hospitals, payment from health insurance now accounts for over 50 percent of income. This means that at the level of the government provider, such as the district or provincial hospital, health insurance revenues can constitute a significant part of the recurrent costs. The positive nature of this new form of financing health care, with direct transfer of funds between the social health insurance system and the public health care providers, obviously has advantages for balanced health system development and gains in the quality of care. An obvious expectation would be that when health insurance revenues account for the major part of provider revenue, the understanding of the importance of health insurance increases and there is more public support to strengthen the system.

The question is how do provider revenues from health insurance actually increase? There is an urgent need to control VHI expenditures on health care, as analyses of expenditure reflect considerable abuse. De facto this means that there is a need to monitor and control the proportion of provider revenue from this source. Essentially, the public health system and the providers have to understand that any increase in the proportion of revenues should be linked to an increase in the number of insured persons, rather than an increase in the volume and nature of services generated. The social health insurance system simply cannot afford to increase membership until the provider initiated abuse is curtailed. The providers also have to realize that the increase in the number of insured persons will be promoted by the delivery of appropriate services, in visibly improved patient conditions.

Health insurance development in Vietnam is no longer a policy question of how to finance health care. The government has adopted health insurance as a national policy, and sees the contributions of the population as a long-term approach to reducing government health care expenditure and reaching stability in financing health care. The establishment of VHI provincial offices in all provinces, and the registration of almost 10 million insured persons within six years of operation may be seen as remarkable. The future extension of coverage poses a set of challenges which require a strengthening of partnerships and understanding at central and provincial levels, and between the different government and private partners involved. Perhaps the major conclusion of the development to date takes the form of a question: at what stage should legislation to achieve universal health insurance be prepared and implemented? The process of starting with a decree rather than law afforded a period of experimentation, flexibility and design of health insurance scheme elements to suit local factors. Until the appropriate legislation can be drafted, passed into law and implemented, there are many areas for further improvement as well as possibilities to test options, in both the compulsory and voluntary components of the VHI scheme. It is important that these challenges be taken on rapidly. There are already private for-profit health insurance initiatives trying to garner the high-wage salaried sector, which would limit the chances to strengthen the VHI fund. As noted above, this high salary population is crucial for fund viability. It is even more important for equity.

Zimbabwe

Background. The slow but steady growth of the Commercial and Industrial Medical Aid Society (CIMAS) in Zimbabwe has not attracted much attention to date. This is unfortunate, as the roots and evolution of this scheme have valuable lessons for developing countries going through various forms of transition. CIMAS first launched operations in October 1945 covering all enterprises which were members of the Chamber of Commerce (Chaora, 1994). The establishment of CIMAS in fact followed the operation of in-house company schemes to cover the health expenditures of select company staff. This development of CIMAS as a mutual aid society was done to enable the sharing of risks, funds and administration. The administrative structure created was later able to undertake the extension of coverage to all employees of the major industrial sector and parastatal companies, with the exception of civil servants.

The contributions for salaried employed were income related and usually shared equally between employers and workers. From the beginning, CIMAS enabled the enrollment of the self-employed, as individuals or as families, on a flat rate contribution basis on collective rather than individual risk for population groups. From the beginning, the national income tax authorities accepted that this health insurance mechanism was an income distribution instrument and therefore the contributions were tax deductible. This continuation has come under review in the framework of economic structural adjustment in Zimbabwe but has not been changed.

Since its inception, CIMAS has operated as a non-profit mutual society. Supervised by a Board, it has had relative freedom in adapting to market forces by introducing changes into existing schemes as well as creating new schemes to meet the needs of specific population sectors. CIMAS has grown significantly in membership, through almost two decades of civil unrest before independence, and through the ensuing period of slow economic growth in Zimbabwe. Assisted by the nature of its operations, CIMAS was relatively successful in its cost containment measures, mainly designed to counter the disadvantages of the fee-for-service provider payment system. The cost containment included limited undertakings to directly provide selected health care services (such as laboratory services), changes in benefits to include selected preventive services and through annual negotiations with Zimbabwe Medical Association to renew contractual agreements regarding fee schedules with both public and private health care providers. These fee schedules are now calculated according to a Zimbabwe Relative Value Scale (ZRVS), which takes into account the time aspects of the health professionals and updated cost estimates, for a defined list of procedures. The contractual agreements are made with public health care providers, private non-profit and for-profit providers (the latter are mainly hospitals, group practice clinics and diagnostic facilities) as well as individual private practitioners. The contractual agreements serve as a de facto accreditation mechanism.

Government policy regarding health care financing following independence should be noted. The first measure after independence in 1980 was to introduce free health care for all citizens earning less than a defined amount, set at slightly less than the minimum wage at the time. Patients earning above the amount were supposed to pay according to income levels. The policy was applied to government hospitals as well as government-assisted health facilities, which meant the religious mission hospitals and facilities run by local authorities. However, in practice, the fees collected amount to 2 - 3 percent of the hospital budgets, and this yield was in fact lower than the costs of collecting the fees (Sikipa, 1991). A major reason was the difficulty in means testing patients and de facto, care given in public hospitals and clinics remained free of charge for most patients. This resulted in congestion, long waiting times and shortages of medicines. Pressure from workers in salaried employment came from the desire to have access to the private (non-profit as well as for-profit health care facilities) rather than from increased labor organization. The pressure on employers was further increased when fees in government hospitals were increased significantly in 1992, with tertiary care fees increasing by as much as 80 percent.

The negative health care and political results of these attempts at cost recovery in Ministry of Health hospitals were very quickly recognized, and the policy of high user charges was reversed. A series of consultations, mainly with bilateral donor agencies, were started to find alternatives, and the conclusion was to develop social health insurance through a National Health Insurance Commission. There was certainly less pressure to implement government-sponsored health insurance given the significant coverage achieved by CIMAS. At various stages in the formulation of the policy on health insurance as the optimal health care financing method, CIMAS offered to undertake prime responsibility for larger scale implementation of a compulsory health insurance law. This could have facilitated implementation, as the necessary registration and contribution collection functions were already in place in all parts of the country.

In the same period, essentially beginning in the mid-1980s, the government made serious attempts to increase the general taxation base and to generate funds through heavy import duties and restrictions in foreign currency exchange. The National Health Insurance Project was temporarily dropped because of the recent cost of living increases, and the unpopularity of further statutory deductions, particularly as violent labor unrest followed large-scale retrenchment of workers. From 1996 there has been renewed activity, mainly in the form of studies funded by bilateral donors. In the meantime, the government established a National Social Security Commission to set up a national pension scheme for all salaried workers. So far, there has been no formal linkage between this commission and the national health insurance development efforts.

Extension of coverage. In terms of innovations in the extension of coverage, CIMAS developed schemes for low income workers, taking into consideration sensitive political issues in labor policies following independence (Abel-Smith 1992, Bailey 1993). With independence in 1980, the political economy created pressures on companies to provide uniform benefits among workers in all racial groups in areas related to salary, job status as well as welfare benefits. CIMAS had in fact followed a multiracial membership policy since 1969 but few blacks were covered prior to independence. At that time, the insured population of 220,000 workers were mainly from the white communities which had access to information and the benefits of health insurance. By 1992, membership was over 600,000, and black membership accounted for 72 percent of the total membership as compared to 7 percent in 1980. The number of insured in 1992 represented around 40 percent of the estimated 1,500,000 workers in the formal sector, in a total national population of 10.4 million. CIMAS now has five schemes, covering different population groups for an increased range of services, and with a total membership of 404,000 household heads in 1998. In addition, CIMAS operations in-house schemes for two large companies and the students of two universities.

By 1994, three fairly comprehensive schemes had been developed for low income earners, to complement the two existing schemes for middle and higher income salaried workers as well as self-employed and non-economically active individual schemes. Contributions to each of the schemes are flat amounts, remitted voluntarily through the employers or the insured persons. The extent of sharing between employers and workers is left to the individual employers. The major difference between these and the previous schemes is that inpatient benefits are limited to services provided by public and mission hospitals, but not private for-profit hospitals. The health care benefits reflect a comprehensive approach with primary health care as the foundation and referrals for other non-emergency services.

The General Package scheme is the most comprehensive and provides access to most health services. The monthly premium at the end of 1998 was the equivalent of US$ 6.64 for adults and US$ 3.41

for dependent minors, with the possibility of membership for other dependents of the household at the adult contribution rate. These are generally elderly dependent parents. The benefits cover full payment in public hospitals and clinics for outpatient and inpatient care, according to the ZRVS. Benefits include payment in full for private general practitioner care, prescribed drugs, blood transfusions, ambulance services, home nursing care and ancillary diagnostic services. Dental care, family planning, rehabilitation services (physiotherapy, speech and occupational therapy as well as prostheses), social work, clinical psychology, psychiatry and treatment outside the country are covered up to specific amounts. By 1998, membership in the General Package Scheme totalled 59,110 insured persons, following an increase of 21 percent in membership from 1994.

The Primary Care Scheme is targeted at low-income workers, such as shopfloor employees. The monthly premium was the equivalent of US$ 2.82 for individuals covered. The full cost of medical expenses are met, provided treatment is given by government doctors (including specialists) and dentists and by private general practitioners. The benefits cover full costs of the same range of services as the General Package, but have lower amounts as maximum limitations on rehabilitation services, prostheses and appliances. The number of consultations with private general practitioners is now limited to 12 visits per person per year, while there are no limitations on the number of visits to public (government and mission) facilities, nurses and maternity related care. Ambulatory prescription drugs have an annual limit, while drugs supplied to patients in public hospitals are paid in full. The limitation on the number of visits to general practitioners (which can be lifted on appeal in regard to the specific case) were made following abuse by beneficiaries on this package. The abuse included trading in membership cards, enabling non-insured persons to have access to the general practitioners. CIMAS internal analysis showed that members with this package had the highest rate of general practitioner visits per person.

Between 1994 and 1997, membership increased from 62,500 to 76,500, but then decreased by over 10 percent to 68,400 in 1998. There are several explanations for this decrease. One is the reaction to the limitation of general practitioner visits applied in 1997. Another is the significant retrenchment of workers in 1998 linked to the national economy. In that year, several large textile factories closed or transferred operations to neighboring countries where foreign exchange conditions were more favorable. On the positive side, some members in the Primary Scheme were able to upgrade to the General scheme.

The Basic Scheme was the last to be introduced, starting in 1994. The scheme targets mainly domestic workers. With a monthly premium of the equivalent of US$ 0.67 per member, the scheme covers the full costs of care at government, municipal and mission hospitals and clinics throughout the country. This package does not cover private general practitioner care. Prescribed drugs dispensed by the public facilities are paid in full, while the limits on dental care, blood transfusions, rehabilitation and ambulance services have lower annual caps than the Primary and General Schemes. By 1998, the Basic Scheme had over 27,000 members, some of whom had downgraded from the Primary Scheme when they lost salaried jobs in 1997.

The growth in all three low-income worker schemes has been impressive, with membership in all three schemes reaching over 161,000 insured persons in 1998. CIMAS believes that the major hindrance to growth is that social health insurance is not yet understood. The most common misconception of those that have joined is that every medical care bill will be taken care once they become members. As need arises, there are disappointments and drop outs. Membership is voluntary, and employers who encounter dissatisfaction among covered workers may be quick to stop paying. With the dramatic increase in HIV/AIDS patients in Zimbabwe, CIMAS has had to contend with a new and serious problem. Over 25 percent of the adult population in Zimbabwe are HIV positive. CIMAS does not exclude such individuals from membership, but none of the three schemes include care in private nursing homes, to which many terminal AIDS cases are ultimately referred. Home care is covered only in the General Scheme.

Most of the efforts to attract new employers and new members were carried out through a Marketing Division set up in 1988. The approach taken by CIMAS in extending coverage to low income populations was to enroll all individuals who showed interest and to offer comprehensive rather than fragmented packages. Caps were placed only on ancillary services and drugs, in which abuse is most likely to occur. As opposed to Vietnam, coverage of dependents of the low income workers was encouraged, as selective individual membership was seen as another potential area of abuse.

Conclusions

The first part of this chapter showed that workers themselves, through mutual societies and later labor as employers associations, were the main driving force in the initial development of social health insurance. The introduction of social health insurance and the extent of coverage in developing countries came from different sources, and in fact did not benefit from active and positive labor and employer initiatives. To some extent, it is unfortunate that the positive developments in health insurance development were not better coordinated with the traditional tripartite partners and overall social security development. While we can learn from the process, it is difficult to predict the potential influence of labor and employer forces, if they could be stimulated to be concerned with the development of social health insurance today. The employment environment is vastly different. There are also obvious shifts in the meaning of solidarity at all levels. It would be inappropriate to expect a significant revival change in solidarity in an era when demographic changes reduce solidarity even at the family level.

The review of recent innovations, in Vietnam and Zimbabwe, demonstrated that the extension of coverage in new and developing health insurance schemes may be linked to a different set of factors, which indeed may be easier to deal with in terms of achieving the targets in the extension of coverage. In broad terms, these factors include the administrative capacity of the health insurance schemes and the parallel development of health services systems with visible improvements in the quality of care.

Administrative capacity denotes more than the ability of a health insurance scheme to function efficiently. The issues which determine the ability of a specific scheme to extend coverage to new populations begin with the ability to make decisions on the one hand, and continue with the ability to carry out the necessary functions to implement the decisions. One of the problems encountered in extending voluntary health insurance coverage in the initial stage was unfamiliarity with a decision- making process at the provincial or decentralized level. As a new health insurance scheme matures, these problems are detected and can be solved. However, this will only happen if there are clear guidelines for decision making and tools for their implementation at the decentralized level. An example of such a decision is the approach to the enrollment of new members. In Vietnam, the decision to facilitate anything more frequent than annual registration and contribution collection took several years. Provisions for registration throughout the year and monthly contribution collection are still not in place is most provinces. In Zimbabwe, a social marketing approach was used from the very beginning, allowing for anyone to join at any time, and pay contributions on a monthly basis.

The compliance problem is more complex, and the importance of this area cannot be overestimated. Apart from the national level target to reach universal coverage, every health insurance scheme is concerned with the negative effects of low compliance. In the first instance, the viability of the scheme will depend to a large extent on the economic strength of the fund. Some health insurance schemes have taken an approach that good investment in the contribution revenues can compensate for low compliance. This approach is not compatible with social health insurance, particularly in a developing country and for low-income workers. Clearly, all revenues from the fund, after deduction for reasonable administrative costs, are needed to provide better health services in an under-funded health care system. Low compliance, as in Vietnam, means that while the majority of low salaried civil servants are covered, only a minority of higher paid private sector workers are covered. The financial viability of the scheme therefore suffers, undermining the advantages of having one scheme for both public and private sectors.

However, any assessment of compliance begins with the administration of the scheme, and its capacity to obtain and analyze the necessary information. The social health insurance scheme requires access to a reasonably complete list of enterprises or individuals who would be covered by compulsory insurance. If the scheme is part of a broad social insurance system, it may be in a more favorable situation regarding access to this information. If not, the scheme needs to identify other appropriate sources, including the regular purchasers of public utilities in a given area. The solutions to compliance problems obviously involve more than administrative capacity. There are misconceptions regarding limitations of benefits in the form of maximum amount covered for any specific service. Along with co-payments, these measures make the schemes less attractive.

The basic problem, however, is the lack of sanctions, either because the scheme is voluntary, or because the sanctions require the backing of legislation rather than decrees.

Social marketing and flexibility in administrative functions to make health insurance "user friendly" need to be backed by parallel developments in the health care system. Even if new and significantly high charges are the alternative at the time that health care is used, the insured have to identify visibly in the availability and quality of care through their regular contributions. Continued long waiting times and the lack of prescribed medicines are major areas of complaint, regardless of any abuse by the insured or providers. Finally, efforts to extend coverage of social health insurance need to recognize the expectations and obligations of the target populations. Healthy adults workers may make infrequent use of services, and need to know that they have the security of other mechanisms in cases of work injury or motor vehicle accidents if these are not covered by the health insurance scheme. The working population is more likely to be concerned with access to health care and expenditure for their dependents, who are also likely to have greater needs. In order to ultimately enable universal coverage, the extension of coverage therefore needs to be carried out with a clear understanding of the initiatives, with coordination between old and new partners and with a comprehensive approach to the health of the family.

References

Abel-Smith, B. 1992. "Health insurance in developing countries: lessons from experience." *Health Policy and Planning*: 7 (3) 215-226.

Atim, C. 1994. "In Search of self-reliance: The case of grass-roots social movements in Africa." Brussels, World Solidarity, 1994.

Bailey, C., van Ginneken, W., and van der Hoeven, R. 1993. "Structural change and adjustment in Zimbabwe: Report of an ILO Mission to Zimbabwe." International Labour Organization, ILO.

Chaora, M. 1994. Report presented at the WHO Inter-regional Consultative Meeting on Health Insurance, Seoul.

Chaora, M. 1999. Private communication.

Carrin G., Sergent, F. and Murray M. 1993. *Towards a framework for health insurance development in Hai Phong, Viet Nam.* WHO, Geneva: Macroeconomics, Health and Development Series, No.12.

Perrot, J. and Sergent, F. 1991. *Rapport de mission auprès du Ministere de la Santé* (WHO Report), Hanoi, Vietnam.

Robb, C., and Zhang. 1998. "Social Aspects of the Crisis: Perceptions of Poor Communities in Thailand." Paper prepared for Thailand's Social Investment Project of the World Bank, Mimeo.

Ron, A., Carrin, G., and Tien, V.T. 1998. "Viet Nam: The development of national health insurance." *International Social Security Review*, Vol.51, 3/98.

Sikipa, G. 1991. "Cost Recovery in Ministry of Health Hospitals—Republic of Zimbabwe—Policy issues and developments in past year." International Health Policy Program, Carnegie Foundation Report, 1991.

Tran Van Tien. 1996. "Report of medical supervision activities and health care expenditure in the first six months of 1996." VHI Central Office, Hanoi.

Weinert, P. 1991. *Foreign Female Domestic Workers: Help wanted!* International Labour Organization, Geneva: International Migration for Employment, Working Paper No. 50, ISBN 92-2-107907-4.

Vietnam Health Insurance. 1998. Reports of studies carried out through the WHO Health Insurance Development Project, VHI Office, Hanoi.

3

Health Protection for Informal Sector Workers: New Approaches to a Long-Standing Problem

W. van Ginneken *

In most countries of the developing and developed world, informal sector workers remain an important part of the workforce. This is contrary to the perceived wisdom in development economics which had assumed that with continuing economic growth more and more workers would become part of the formal sector. At the same time, in most developing countries structural adjustment measures over the past 10-15 years have forced many governments to cut down on social services, including access to health services. While formal sector workers often enjoy health protection, in the form of access to health services in general as well as to safety and health measures at work in particular, such protection has generally not been extended to the large majority of informal sector workers.

The purpose of this chapter is to document and discuss various aspects of an integrated approach to health protection, i.e., the financing and organization of preventive, promotive and curative health services, by and for informal sector workers. This chapter will analyze the various reasons why the extension of formal sector social security schemes has not taken place, and it will then look into the various options for organizing health protection for and/or by informal sector workers. A new health protection approach was

---

* With many thanks to David Dror for his helpful comments.

tested by means of a pilot experience undertaken in Dar es Salaam within the context of ILO's Informal Sector Interdepartmental Project (Kiwara, 1999). The model of health-care delivery applied in this project is based on the local capacity of the informal sector operators to undertake low-cost improvements at the workplace level, to prevent injuries and diseases, and to enhance access to health care through the introduction of a self-financed health insurance scheme.

This chapter will start with introducing the concept of health protection and with examining the role of informal sector workers' associations in an increasingly private sector market for health services. The second section will examine why personal social protection coverage is low in the informal sector, and the third section will review the role of group-based health insurance as a means to extend curative health protection to informal sector workers. The fourth section will discuss various ways to promote health at work, whereas the last section will review some policy conclusions.

Health Protection, Markets and Informal Sector Worker's Associations

The health of informal sector workers and their families is affected by their living conditions, as well as by the organization and financing of health services. What households can do is determined, to a great extent, by their income, knowledge, level of schooling as well as by the status of women. Especially in the poorest countries, government policies and actions that accelerate income growth and reduce poverty make it possible for people to afford better diets, healthier living conditions and better health care. Policies to expand educational opportunities, particularly for girls, help households achieve healthier lives by increasing their access to information and their ability to make good use of it. The same goes for policies that work to ensure effective and accessible health services for all. When all these policies are combined, they can create a virtuous cycle in which reduction of poverty and improvements in health reinforce each other (IBRD, 1993).

Actions on safety and health as well as on health insurance have to fit into this larger framework of policy actions. In addition, they have to take account of the fact that in the informal sector the distinction between working and living conditions is often blurred and that policy actions have to be designed so as to fit in with the complete work and life situation of informal sector workers and their families. Their income and work situation is characterized by great insecurity: they are often obliged to live from one day to the next. Informal sector workers generally have a short-term planning horizon, since they are not in control of most factors affecting their work and life.

The Concept of Health Protection

In general, health protection can be defined as "any kind of collective measure or activity designed to ensure that members of society attain and maintain an adequate level of health." Such measures and activities can range from prevention and promotion to curative and rehabilitative health care. In addition, they can be organized and/or financed by the state and groups of society but carried out by public or private sector health care providers.

Historically, there was some advantage for the state in organizing and financing health programs that strike against health problems of entire populations or population subgroups. Their objective is to prevent disease or injury and to provide information on self-cure and on the importance of seeking care. Public health programs generally work in three ways:

- they deliver specific public health services, such as immunization;

- they promote healthy behavior in areas, such as diet and nutrition, family planning and reducing abuse of alcohol, tobacco and drugs; and

- they promote healthy environments at home (water and sanitation), at work (safety and health), and in the physical and human surroundings (air, water, traffic).

According to a recent World Bank publication on health financing (Schieber and Maeda, 1997), public health services should be financed publicly. Personal health services which also have collective benefits should be publicly subsidized, while personal health services can either be publicly or privately financed. Health insurance is considered the preferred vehicle for financing personal health services and has indeed been implemented. However, the informal sector has to a large extent been excluded. Informal risk pooling schemes, often sponsored by local governments and voluntary groups, are considered viable mechanisms in poor urban and rural areas.

Many low-income countries have seen long-term declines in (relative) public health expenditure, so that they can no longer guarantee free access to quality personal health services. So greater scope for private sector provision has been created for households who can afford such services. This was felt quite dramatically in a country, such as Tanzania, which decided in 1991 to abolish the state monopoly in health provision (Kiwara, 1999). Even traditionally public health services, such as water supply and sanitation, are now increasingly produced by enterprises in the formal and informal sectors. For example in Dar es Salaam a neighborhood-based sanitation service was developed using modernized technology and operated by informal sector enterprises (Muller and Rijnsburger, 1996).

The Role of Informal Sector Workers' Associations

In principle, informal sector workers are occupied in (micro-) enterprises with the following characteristics (ILO, 1994):

- the owner is personally liable for gains and losses (the enterprise is not registered as a commercial enterprise);

- absence of full and written accounts; the enterprise has less than 10 continuous employees.

But apart from informal enterprises there are also informal labor relations which means the absence of written labor contracts. Such informality does not only affect wage earners and other groups such as home workers in the informal sector, but also casual laborers who work directly or indirectly—for formal sector enterprises.

Informal sector workers do in many cases organize themselves in order to achieve some benefits for themselves and/or to have greater impact on institutions and authorities that affect their conditions. Their main priority is generally to secure access to capital (credit) and land (stability of tenure). They may also be interested in organizing joint access to productive inputs, such as technology, training and business services. Finally, some of these associations also organize access to social services such as health and education as well as the financing of social security contingencies, including health care. ILO experiences in various parts of the world (Aryee, 1996) have shown informal sector workers can also be interested in organizing safety and health services at work.

The analysis of these experiences as well as those from other countries shows that there are three fundamental requirements for the setting up of successful social health provision and insurance schemes, on a collective risk-pooling basis.

1. the existence of an association based on trust;

2. a basic management and administration capacity for, among other things, collecting contributions and providing benefits;

3. access to expertise in health care organization.

There are various types of groups that organize informal sector workers. Some associations or organizations are directly managed by the informal sector workers themselves, such as producer and employer organizations, cooperatives and credit associations. Other groups of informal sector workers benefit from the services of intermediate carriers such as trade unions, NGOs and private insurance companies. The latter are generally private non-profit health insurance schemes.

Recent activities organized by, and for, informal sector workers are generally based on a comprehensive concept of development and social protection (ILO-SAAT, 1996). Organizations such as NGOs and cooperatives have a good understanding of the particular needs and priorities of their client groups and have developed with them institutions and policies that are quite different from what the government is used to and/or can cope with. In the social field NGO action integrates the traditional social protection measures with complementary measures in the field of (primary) health care, child care, housing and targeted social action. In the economic field, more security can be achieved through self-help and self-employment, resulting in an enhancement of income and creation of productive assets. This not only helps to reduce, to some extent, the need and cost of conventional social security measures available, but also makes a positive economic impact by enabling the poor to actively participate in and contribute to the economy of the nation.

The opportunities for informal (sector) workers to organize themselves generally depend on the area they work and on their employment status. The degree of organization among informal sector workers is, therefore, dependent on the following broad characteristics (van Ginneken, 1996):

- *Urban/rural.* Urban informal workers tend to be more heterogeneous, so that they are likely to find it more difficult to establish associations among themselves.

- *Self-employed/wage earner.* Self-employed workers generally have higher incomes and are better organized than wage earners, with the result that they are better candidates for successfully organizing themselves in cooperatives or other producer organizations.

- *Resident/transient.* Where people are working and living in a fixed place, they are more likely to build up the necessary trust for setting up joint services. So people working in the street economy of the urban areas or seasonal migrants in the rural areas are less likely to be able to organize themselves.

- *Regular/casual.* There are some regular wage workers in the informal sector who may be covered by compulsory social insurance schemes, which generally cater to workers in the formal sector. Casual workers—both in the formal and informal sectors—are usually not organized in trade unions, and therefore tend to be excluded from statutory social insurance schemes. Given their weak organizational base and the instability of their employment, they are usually not able to set up their own schemes either.

Group-based Schemes Faced with the Market for Health Services

In many developing countries, health care market institutions are not highly developed. As a result, organizational purchasers are a weak force in the market, the quality of health care provided may be low and consumers may be faced with a bewildering number of health care choices (Bennett, 1997).

The disruption of public health services, recent application of user charges and increased availability of private providers pose new problems to the consumers of health services, in particular for informal sector workers who are not used to dealings with private health providers. Informal sector workers can benefit from the intermediation of self-organized and self-financed group-based structures that deal and negotiate with private (and public health providers) on their behalf. Table 3.1 reflects the idea that there are multiple forms of group organizations that cater to health services. It also points to the growing importance and opportunities for group-based schemes and private sector health care provision in a changing market for health services.

Many group- and community-based schemes reviewed by Bennett et al. (1998) act as intermediaries between the individual and the (public or private) provider of primary, secondary or tertiary care. The UMASIDA scheme in Dar es Salaam, for example, shows that the social financing of health care can go in parallel with the provision of health education at work. Another study (Muller and Rijnsburger, 1996) shows that water and sanitation can also be financed and managed by informal sector associations.

In general, the table shows that there is a wide variety of options to the financing (effective demand) and delivery (supply) of health care services. While immunization and the provision of a healthy environment is in principle an activity financed by the (central and local) government, primary health care as well as adequate household, water and sanitation services can be financed by individuals, groups as well as the government.

With regard to the delivery of services, the local government can in principle provide all of them, except tertiary health care which—with immunization and the ambient environment—is mainly the responsibility of the central government. Table 3.1 shows that the private sector can supply an important array of health services, ranging from health education, curative services to water and sanitation facilities.

Table 3.1
Effective Demand and Supply of Health Services

Type of health service	EFFECTIVE DEMAND (financing)			SUPPLY (production)		
	Individual	Group-based	Public goods	Local Government	Central Government	Private sector
Immunization			x	x	x	
Health education		x	x	x		x
Primary health care	x	x	x	x		x
Secondary health care	x	x		x		x
Tertiary health care	x	x			x	x
Water and sanitation	x	x	x	x		x
Ambient environment			x	x	x	

Behind the picture of changing market structures is hidden the changed relationship between the consumers and producers of health services. In the case of the health care market, the mix of demand and supply is determined first of all by quality, and only in second instance by price (Bennett, 1997). As is happening in many social security branches, various components in the provision of benefits can be subcontracted to the private sector through the intermediation of group-based structures. In economic literature this is called the "principal-agency" relationship, where the "principal" is the group-based structure and the "agency" the (private) health providers. The "principal" attempts to steer the "agency" into the desired direction by means of "contracts," such as fee for service, flat rate and capitation fee (Normand and Weber, 1994).

Reasons for Low Personal Health and Social Security Coverage

Informal sector workers have generally been excluded from health insurance provided by statutory national social security schemes. It was found in Tanzania, for example, that such health insurance schemes hardly exist (Kiwara, 1999). Colombia has tried to extend health insurance coverage through the so-called "health solidarity enterprises" that were meant to work on a capitation payment basis (González Posso et al., 1995). However, the extension has reached much fewer people than planned, mainly for the following three reasons. First, there were ideological battles within the Ministry of Health about whether the "demand" or the "supply" of health services should be subsidized. Second, the ministry paid the capitation only for very limited groups of workers. And third, many "solidarity health enterprises" did not always have the managerial capacity to organize a complicated business such as health insurance. In the Philippines, legal extensions were enacted, but for various reasons without much real effect (ILO, 1996). That was the reason behind the decision in 1995 to establish the Philippines Health Insurance Corporation as a separate social health insurance scheme.

In the eyes of many informal sector workers in the Philippines, cooperative social security arrangements are much more user-friendly and flexible, because administrative procedures are simpler, and people are allowed some flexibility in making their contributions. On the other hand, formal social security arrangements usually do not apply and/or are not suitable to informal sector workers for some of the following reasons:

- ignorance about rights and obligations;

- the intermittent working status of most informal sector workers, resulting in low and irregular contributory capacity to social security;

- the complicated administrative procedures required from beneficiaries (filling out forms; collection of contributions; documents to be produced).

In some developing countries the process of economic growth has resulted in the transfer of a large part of the labor force to the formal sector. In addition, in these countries the government had—and used—sufficient resources to subsidize the extension of the formal social insurance schemes. This has been the case in various countries from East and Southeast Asia. The most striking example is the Republic of Korea, which achieved universal health insurance coverage in 1989 within about 15 years of the commencement of compulsory medical insurance in 1977 (Park, 1992).

However in most developing countries structural adjustment policies have contributed to a decline in the—often small—percentage of the working population in the formal sector. The successive waves of structural adjustment programs have also led to wage cuts in the public and private sectors, thereby eroding the financial base of statutory social insurance schemes. Simultaneously, many such schemes in developing countries have suffered from bad management, partly because of some inappropriate use of social security funds as loans to fund government activities, which has often strongly reduced the trust of members in the scheme.

In addition, structural adjustment programs have often resulted in severe cuts in social budgets, leading to the deterioration of public primary health care services in most low-income developing countries. The ideal solution is to publicly finance access to basic health care, but since this is not likely to happen in the foreseeable future, there is inevitably a strong demand for group arrangements to finance and organize these social services. In this situation, it is usually more efficient to be part of a group insurance scheme than to have to face health and education expenditures individually (van Ginneken, 1999a). This is particularly true for health care, in which the time of need and the scope and cost of services are usually unpredictable.

Generally speaking, the principal social protection priorities for informal sector workers are related to more immediate needs and to some possible catastrophic events, such as (van Ginneken, 1999b):

- improving the effectiveness of household health care expenditure;

- death, survivor and disability benefits;

- regularizing expenditure on basic education;

- maternity and childcare benefits.

The total contribution rate for statutory social insurance is often 20 percent or more of the total payroll. Formal sector wage workers share these contributions with their employers. However, self-employed workers are often not prepared to pay the full (workers' and employers') contribution by themselves, and they have various ways to escape compliance. In addition, they have irregular income patterns, since their earnings are often dependent on the business cycle and various product and services markets. Other informal sector workers, such as casual and seasonal wage earners are also excluded from statutory social insurance schemes, since they tend to have low and irregular earning patterns. Their employment depends on the availability of jobs in specific periods. When there is no work, employment is immediately terminated, and hence incomes are lost.

The fundamental reason for low social security coverage in developing countries is therefore that many workers outside the formal sector are not able or willing to contribute a relatively high percentage of their incomes to finance social security benefits that do not meet their immediate priority needs. Since statutory social insurance schemes are compulsory and do not generally allow workers (or their employers) to insure for some benefits and not others, they perpetuate a situation in which the majority of workers remain excluded. Moreover, given the extent of exclusion, it is understandable that workers within such schemes are not willing to extend coverage to workers outside the scheme who—even if they were interested in joining—have lower contributory capacity and would have to be supported with cross-subsidies. As far as self-employed persons are concerned, this suggests that compulsory coverage may be feasible only through special schemes.

The Role of Group-based Health Insurance

Various self-employed and informal sector workers have set up their own schemes in order to meet their priority social protection needs. The mechanism used in these schemes is generally the provision of mutual support through the pooling of resources based on the principles of insurance, help being extended to those in need within the overall framework of certain basic regulatory conditions. In this system, it is the group itself that decides on the size and the source of contributions that group members are meant to make. The collection and management of contributions—as well as the disbursement of benefits—are again matters for the group to consider and arrange.

In a recent article, Dror and Jacquier (1999) set out the concept of micro-insurance and its basic tenets: (i) the insurance is autonomously managed by groups and units at the local level; and—ideally—(ii) the local unit is structured in such a way as to link up with multiple small area- and occupation-based units into larger structures that can enhance both the insurance function and the support structures needed for improved governance. Such local micro-insurance structures have the advantages of cohesion, direct participation and low administrative costs.

As noted earlier, health insurance is often felt to be the most urgent social protection priority by informal sector workers (see, for example, Kamuzora, 1999). As shown in some of the recent literature (Atim, 1998; ILO-SAAT, 1996; Bennett et al., 1998), informal sector health insurance schemes often cover high-cost, low-frequency events (inpatient hospital care), or low-cost, high-frequency events (primary health care), and in some cases a mix between them. They are designated as Type I and Type II schemes respectively in table 3.2. The frequency of service utilization and possibilities for cost control are different in the two types of scheme.

Hospital-based insurance schemes covering hospital costs have been proposed (see, for example Shaw and Griffin, 1995) as one of the strategies for generating additional revenues for health financing. These schemes have generally been set up in a context of reduced government or donor financing, and are basically aimed at putting hospital financing on a sound footing. Some of these schemes face high and rising costs because they suffer from adverse selection, and patients tend to enroll when they know that they will need hospital care.

Table 3.2
Two Ends of the Health Cost Risk-Sharing Spectrum

Type of scheme	Type I	Type II
Costs insured	Inpatient hospital care	Primary health care Cost
Cost per intervention	High	Low
Frequency of utilization	Low	High
Ownership	Hospital	Community or association
Coverage	District	Community or association
Basis for premium setting	Actuarial study	Ability to pay

Source: Adapted from Bennett et al., 1998, p. 10.

In addition, hospital-based schemes often lead to over-prescription and over-provision of services. Finally, they provide relatively high-cost primary and secondary health care services.

Governments in many developing countries claim to provide free or subsidized access to basic health care for low-income families. But in practice, many workers—even those with incomes under the poverty line—can spend between 5 and 10 percent of their income on health services (Jain, 1999), so that they are potential candidates for participating in health insurance schemes. As a result, informal sector workers prefer to contribute to micro-insurance health schemes focused on the provision of primary and some secondary health care services for which they face relatively small but periodical expenses. These schemes usually have low population coverage.

The main advantage of micro-health insurance schemes is that they improve health expenditure efficiency or the relation between quality and cost of health services. There are basically three reasons why participants in such schemes would prefer group schemes to individual spending and financing (van Ginneken, 1998):

1. by regular contributions, the problem of debt brought about by high medical bills can be alleviated;

2. the financial power of the group may enable administrators to negotiate services of better quality or better value for money from private health care providers; and

3. the group may be willing to spend on preventive and health promotion activities so as to keep down the cost of medical services.

The experience with the UMASIDA (Health fund for informal sector workers) scheme in Dar es Salaam (Kiwara, 1999) confirms that access to primary and some secondary health care is often the first priority for informal sector workers schemes. The second priority is access to inpatient hospital care, which can be organized in a special insurance arrangement. Focusing on primary services first has the additional advantage that better access to primary health care services will reduce the demand for hospital services (see advantage 3 above). On the other hand, the ORT Health Plus Scheme (OHPS) in the Philippines shows the financial viability and health care advantages of comprehensive benefits, with a strong primary health care base.

Sustainability and Coverage

In their review of rural risk-sharing strategies in health, Bennett, Creese and Monash (1998) note that there are several threats to the scope for raising revenues through health insurance schemes. The threats include:

- the small scale of the majority of schemes examined;

- adverse selection leading to progressively smaller risk pools and higher costs;

- heavy administrative structures and costs in some schemes.

These three threats are clearly interrelated, because the heavy administrative structure and costs are often the result of the scheme's small scale. In addition, the small scale of most of the schemes is reinforced by the problem of adverse selection. So one key issue is to define under what conditions health insurance schemes can be sustainable and/or replicable.

A health insurance scheme could be called sustainable when it is able to deliver an appropriate level of health benefits to the client group for an extended period of time (Henriques, 1994). Health insurance schemes have *organizational sustainability* when they are embedded within an organizational or networking structure which

- possess a high level of *organizational legitimacy* with national and international interest groups, i.e., when they are perceived as serving an important need.

- possess the *managerial capacity* to serve the need in a cost-effective, professional and accountable manner. This means that the organization must have the vision, commitment and organizational capability to continue to remain relevant, and mobilize stakeholders and resources. This dimension covers various aspects: leadership, managerial capability and systems, staff motivation, organizational culture, organizational commitment to health provision, etc.

Technical sustainability refers to the degree to which the scheme is capable of continuing, and possibly improving, the *quality of services* and also extending benefits and coverage. This dimension covers such aspects as technical ability and knowledge of management, staff and health providers, and ability to monitor evolving client needs.

Financial sustainability refers to the degree to which the scheme is able to generate adequate income to cover the associated costs. The income can be generated from user contributions, outside support as well as government subsidies, as long as they are available over longer periods of time and in a predictable way. These aspects of sustainability cover issues such as cost structure, perceived value creation for clients, ability and willingness of participants to pay, and demand for services from other organizations.

Replicating Group-based Health Insurance Schemes on a Wider Scale

There are various characteristics on the basis of which work- and residence-based groups can organize themselves for the provision of health protection. People can organize themselves because they share the same occupation, live in the same area or belong to the same gender, cultural or religious group, for example. Each of these characteristics has its own advantages and disadvantages with regard to group factors such as trust, leadership, as well as financial and organizational capacity. These characteristics also have a major impact on the extent and speed with which self-financed health insurance schemes can be replicated, or adapted to meet local conditions.

In most countries, work-based organizations have been at the origin of statutory social insurance programs. Informal sector workers—to the extent that they are organized at all—are principally organized in occupation- or sector-based associations and cooperatives. Their first priority is to improve their economic base in terms of credit, marketing and production technology. Once that is ensured, their organizations can often constitute a foundation for the establishment of contributory social and health protection schemes. This is also frequently true for women's organizations, whose purpose often includes raising consciousness with regard to the position of women in the family, work and society. Some of these organizations have set up savings and/or credit bodies which significantly improve the chances of successfully organizing social and health protection schemes.

It seems likely that women are generally more interested in and committed to the provision of health care and education to their family, rather than in occupation-based (and often male-dominated) schemes, which tend to consider disability and survivor pensions as a greater priority. Most work-based schemes are characterized by a high level of group cohesion, but they take a long time to mature. These differences in source of initiative obviously hinder the replication of such schemes.

Organizations based on the place of residence are usually less cohesive, since they may not be interested in the participation of poor people, given their weak financial base (Weinberger and Jütting, 1999). This may be different in the case of rural areas, where communities are often close-knit, and people have similar financial resources. At the area (district) level the social cohesion is likely to be even lower, but the quality of local government strongly influences whether some form of consensus, incentives and accountability can be established. The area-based approach is very suitable for social health care financing, since it can take into account the provision of not only curative but also preventive and promotional activities. In addition, participation by local government can also increase the extent and speed of replication of pilot experiences. In addition, local health insurance schemes can help to relieve some of the pressures on the budget of the Ministry of Health. This idea was worked out in India by Hsiao and Sen (1995) who proposed to manage and finance some primary and secondary health care services through local communities, particularly in the rural areas.

Improving Health at Work

Workers in the informal sector are subjected to the many health hazards that are common to all urban poor families, including pollution, unsanitary living conditions and poor nutrition. Houses which double as workplaces are small and poorly constructed with inadequate light and ventilation. It is often difficult to make a distinction between the health problems which are caused by these conditions and those that are caused specifically from work. Often poor health that may be caused by the general environment in urban poor areas is aggravated by harmful working conditions. For example, a workers' eyesight may be failing due to poor nutrition, and the condition is aggravated by working with poor lighting.

In the informal sector poor working practices and poor working conditions are interrelated. Hazardous working conditions not only harm informal sector workers' health but also decrease their productivity and income. While hazards will vary according to occupation, the most prevalent problems are: poor lighting; lack of ventilation; excessive heat; poor housekeeping; inadequate work space; inadequate working tools, protective equipment and work-space design; awkward postures which induce physical strain and fatigue; exposure to hazardous chemicals and dusts; and long hours of work. Working at home can create additional problems when work and living arrangements interfere with each other and lead to a generally disorderly situation, both for work and for family life.

Various studies have shown that informal sector workers are often under great stress, fatigue and dissatisfaction, which seriously affects their health and can express itself in conditions, such as ulcers and high blood pressure. A study on Colombia for example (González Posso et al., 1995) shows that the physical and emotional stress is highest for informal sector workers on the street, because they are most directly aggressed by traffic, competitors, pedestrians and possibly law enforcement officials. In Dar es Salaam (Kiwara, 1999) the three main health problems are malaria as well as gastro-intestinal and respiratory problems.

In some cases, these diseases have to do directly with the work situation, but they are often also the result of the absence of sanitation and safe water supply and also of a lack of knowledge and/or time to do something about it. In general, informal sector workers are exposed to a host of acute work-related hazards resulting in injuries, chronic conditions, as well as impairments in vision, hearing and mobility. They do not have the benefits of the occupational safety measures and medical attention of the work place.

Targeting Health Promotion on Various Groups of Workers

Efforts to increase the awareness, understanding, and application of ways to improve working conditions can contribute to increased health and safety as well as productivity in the informal sector. But, practically, these efforts need to take into account the realities and limitations in the informal sector. Working conditions are not a priority of informal sector operators. Efforts to address working conditions should therefore be integrated with efforts to increase income levels and security. Simple cost/benefit analysis is an effective tool for concretely showing the impact of occupational health and safety on the productivity of micro-entrepreneurs. Promising approaches promote low-cost ways of improving work tools and workplace designs, maximizing available workspaces to bring about minimal discomfort or pain and exposure to hazardous elements of work.

A particular target group is women in the informal sector. Providing support to women trying to balance multiple roles is critical to concretely improving informal sector working conditions and productivity. Programs should not increase women's burdens by requiring long hours of training but should be designed to fit with women/s schedules and enable women to lessen their working hours. Programs which aim to protect working children and eliminate child labor, increase the availability and quality of child care and improve home-based working conditions are vital to improving the well-being of children (Overy and Piamonte, 1995).

Working conditions in the informal sector cannot be addressed in isolation from living conditions of the urban or rural poor. When basic services and adequate housing are lacking, working conditions are inevitably poor. Efforts to improve working conditions should therefore be integrated with efforts to improve the environment, particularly that of the urban poor communities, including housing, sanitation and access to water and electricity. Improvements in working conditions are a good indicator for improvements in the overall situations of urban poor people.

The informal sector operates largely outside government regulation. Efforts to enforce regulations on working conditions in the informal sector will be costly, difficult to implement and strongly resisted by the informal sector itself. A more effective approach might be to focus on providing guidelines on reasonable working conditions in the informal sector and promoting self-regulation by people's organizations and associations of informal sector workers.

A National Framework for Occupational Safety and Health

There is a great need for national policy framework for the extension of OSH services to the informal sector. In order to achieve any success in the implementation of protective and preventive measures for informal sector workers and their families, all those responsible for OSH should be involved with a clear definition of responsibilities and not only the informal sector operators. Therefore, any initiative in this field should be undertaken in the framework of a national policy to support the informal sector and should involve the relevant authorities and social actors. Such a policy should foresee the need to extend occupational health through primary health care services at the same time that improvements are undertaken at the workplaces through awareness raising and training (Forastieri, Riwa and Swai, 1996).

Informal sector organizations can play a reinforcing role here. They should encourage and undertake organization of informal sector workers, raise awareness on the importance of working conditions and promote self-regulation among their members on maintaining safe and healthy work conditions. Moreover, local government units should prioritize provision of basic services for urban poor communities and support services for women and children.

Innovative approaches and specific methodological tools need to be developed taking into consideration the informal sector characteristics (number of people, widespread poverty, important vulnerable and under-served working population, etc.). To ensure the sustainability of the measures undertaken, they have to be low-cost and practical for the operators. It would also be necessary to identify the links which should be established between the improvement of the working conditions and environment, the protection of the health of the workers and the generation of employment.

Past experiences have shown that any initiative coming from the outside fails as soon as external resources dry up. Impact assessment should be one of the main components of the program in order to adapt it to the real needs of the community, making it affordable and applicable. It should also be kept in mind that the informal sector escapes from the rigidity of formal economic models, being capable of very flexible responses to changes in its overall pattern of economic activity through indigenous initiatives.

Conclusions

Health protection for informal sector workers and their dependants should be seen as an integrated activity, in which all important elements will have to find a place. Health promotion at work as well as at home are critical for improving the health status and income earning capacity of informal sector workers. All the components of a comprehensive spectrum of care should be included: preventive, curative and rehabilitative services.

This chapter argues that health protection strategies should not be considered an affair between governments and individual workers alone, but that intermediate, group-based structures are also necessary to ensure that informal sector workers and their families feel personally concerned and in control of their situation. Incidentally, these forms of group-based organizations are important not only for health protection activities, but also for developmental activities in general. So, another critical condition for the extension of health protection to all is the existence of strong group- and area-based schemes. In countries where national health insurance schemes exist, the support of social partners and other interested parties will be needed.

It is therefore necessary to broaden the health protection partnership and to galvanize the various partners for the design and implementation of a comprehensive health protection policy. Governments, workers and employers constitute core partners, but this partnership must be broadened to promote health protection for low-income workers in self-employment and the informal sector. There is a need for improved linkages between both central and local governments, and between different ministries (social security, labor, health, finance, etc.). An important role will have to be played by local government, by associations that directly represent informal sector workers (such as occupation- and area-based groups, as well as cooperatives, mutual benefit societies and communities) and by intermediary organizations that work on behalf of low-income (wage) workers.

Finally, what is the role of the government? This chapter has shown that, particularly in many low-income developing countries, governments are unable to allocate adequate finances for most health activities. In the absence of universal coverage systems, the optimal solution would be to create structures that can effectively pool the contributions of the informal sector population. The fund created would provide the necessary financing for quality health care, through the underfunded government health services and in cooperation with private and non-government providers. The proposal made by Hsiao and Sen for rural areas in India (1995)—as noted above - goes in the right direction, and should be tried out in pilot projects. Another promising way forward is the development of, and experimentation with, the micro-insurance concept as proposed by Dror and Jacquier (1999). Thus, the government should guarantee at least a minimum amount of resources for primary health care, and support local and group-based schemes with technical cooperation, training and a minimum of regulation, so as to ensure that schemes are managed efficiently and democratically.

References

Aryee, G. 1996. *Promoting productivity and social protection in the urban informal sector. Project implementation report.* The Interdepartmental project on the urban informal sector (Geneva, ILO; IDP. INF/Report).

Atim, C. 1998. *The contribution of mutual health organizations to financing, delivery, and access to health care: Synthesis of research in nine West and Central African countries* (Bethesda, Abt Associates Inc.).

Bennett, S. 1997. "Health markets: defining characteristics." Chapter 6 in Bennett, Sara; McPake, Barbara; and Mills, Anne (eds.) *Private health providers in developing countries: Serving the public interest?* (London, Zed Books).

Bennett, S.; Creese, A.; and Monash, R. 1998. *Health insurance schemes for people outside formal sector employment* (Geneva; WHO Division of Analysis, Research and Assessment; ARA Paper No. 16).

Dror, D.; Jacquier, C. 1999. "Micro-insurance: Extending health insurance to the excluded," in *International Social Security Review* (Geneva, ISSA), Vol. 52, No. 1, pp. 71-97.

Forastieri, V.; Riwa, P; Swai, D. 1996. *Occupational safety and health in the informal sector, Dar es Salaam* (ILO, Geneva; Working Paper for the Interdepartmental Project on the Urban Informal Sector).

van Ginneken, W. 1996. *Social security for the informal sector: Issues, options and tasks ahead* (ILO, Geneva; Working Paper for the Interdepartmental Project on the Urban Informal Sector).

———. (ed.) 1997b. *Social security for the informal sector. Investigating the feasibility of pilot projects in Benin, India, El Salvador and Tanzania* (Geneva; ILO Social Security Department Discussion Paper No. 5).

———. 1998. *Social security for all Indians* (New Delhi, Oxford University Press).

———. (ed.) 1999a. *Social security for the excluded majority. Case studies of developing countries* (Geneva, ILO).

————. 1999b. "Social security for the informal sector. A new challenge for the developing countries," in *International Social Security Review* (Geneva, ISSA) 52(1), pp. 49-69.

González Posso, C. et al. 1995. *El desafío de la informalidad para la seguridad social* (Santa Fé de Bogotá, Corporación Salud y Desarrollo).

Henriques, M. 1994. *What is sustainabiliy in an SED context?* Paper prepared for presentation to the Netherlands Government (ILO, Geneva; unpublished).

Hsiao, W.; and Sen, P. D. 1995. *Cooperative financing for health care in rural India.* Paper presented to the International Workshop on "Health Insurance in India". (Bangalore, IIM, September 20-22).

IBRD, 1993. *World Development Report 1993* (Oxford, Oxford University Press).

ILO. 1994. *Informal sector statistics: Coverage and methodologies* (Geneva, unpublished document by the Interdepartmental Project on the urban informal sector).

ILO. 1996. *Report to the Philippines Government on social protection: Options and recommendations for reform and development.* A Report prepared for the UNDP (Geneva; Report ILO/UNDP/PHI/R.21).

ILO-SAAT. 1996. *Social protection for the unorganized sector in India.* A report prepared for the UNDP under Technical Support Services-1 (New Delhi).

Jain, S. 1999. "Basic social security in India." Chapter 2 in van Ginneken, W. (ed.) *Social security for the excluded majority. Case studies of developing countries* (Geneva, ILO).

Kamuzora, P. 1999. "Extension of formal social security schemes in the United Republic of Tanzania." Chapter 4 in van Ginneken, W. (ed.) *Social security for the excluded majority. Case studies of developing countries* (Geneva, ILO).

Kiwara, A. 1999. "Health insurance for the informal sector in Tanzania." Chapter 5 in van Ginneken, W. (ed.) *Social security for the excluded majority. Case studies of developing countries* (Geneva, ILO).

Muller, M.; and Rijnsburger, J. 1996. "Pit latrines and participation: the MAPET Project in Dar es Salaam," in *Development and Practice* (Oxfam, Oxford), vol. 6 no. 3, pp. 257-261.

Normand, C; and Weber, A. 1994. *Social health insurance. A guidebook for planning* (Geneva, WHO/ILO).

Overy, A.; and Piamonte, D. 1995. *Improving working conditions in the informal sector* (Manila; paper written for the ILO).

Park, T.-W. 1992. "Cost-containment measures in the provision of hospital care under social security health care schemes," in *Report of the ISSA Regional Meeting for Asia and the Pacific on cost-containment measures applied under social security health care schemes* (Geneva, ISSA), Social Security Documentation. Asian and Pacific Series, no. 15.

Ron, A.; and Kupferman, A. 1994. On Bwamanda Scheme, Zaire (page 9).

Schieber, G.; and Maeda, A. 1997. *A Cormudgeon's guide to financing health care in developing countries.* Paper presented to an international conference sponsored by the World Bank on "Innovations in health care financing" (Washington, D.C.).

Shaw, P.; and Griffin, C. 1995. *Financing health care in Sub-Saharan Africa through user fees and insurance* (The World Bank, Washington, D.C.).

Weinberger, K.; and Jütting, J. 1999. *Determinants of participation in community based organizations: Experiences from group based projects in Kashmir and Chad.* (Bonn, Centre for Development Research (ZEF); paper presented to the 11th Annual Meeting on Socio-Economics (SASE), Madison, Wisconsin).

Part 3

Confronting Resource Scarcity: Innovative Strategies

4

Managed Care in the United States: Its History, Forms, and Future

W. Newbrander and R. Eichler

Countries around the world face the challenge of trying to provide more and better-quality health care services with limited resources. One response is the creation of social health insurance programs. Controlling costs and utilization is a necessary adjunct to the introduction of health insurance. Mechanisms to reimburse providers that contain incentives to control utilization and consumer fees to control excessive demand are interventions to control system costs. One form of insurance that is increasingly used to counter inflation is managed care, which provides comprehensive services for its members for a fixed, prepaid fee. Although managed care has different meanings in different countries, the term managed care refers here to the form of health insurance that combines the financing and delivery of health services and integrates elements of cost containment with quality of services.

Managed care has seen dramatic growth as a key element of the health systems in many countries. Elements of managed care have existed in many Latin American countries, with over 60 million people currently enrolled in managed care organizations (MCOs). They continue to grow rapidly in the competitive health insurance markets in Brazil, Chile, and Colombia, as well as in some emerging market countries.1 Principles of managed care are also important in many developed countries, such as the use of the primary care physician as "gatekeeper" in the U.K. Germany now permits MCOs and France's first preferred provider organization was established in 1995.

In the U.S., by 1996 over 25 percent of the population, representing 67 million people, was enrolled in health maintenance organizations (HMOs), a form of managed care (see Figure 4.1). The number of HMOs increased from 174 in 1976 to 651 in 1976 (see Figure 4.2), indicating rapid development of the managed care market. Today over 50 percent of the insured people in the U.S. are enrolled in some form of managed care arrangement.

MCOs are responsible for provision of a comprehensive set of health services to enrolled members in return for a prepaid monthly capitation fee or premium. Much of the growth is a result of managed care bringing together the delivery and financing of health services in cost-effective ways in health systems where most health care services are not managed or financed in a coordinated manner. For example, managed health care programs in the U.S. have had a dramatic impact on shifting specific treatments from an inpatient to an outpatient setting and on reducing the length of stays for hospitalizations.

The trend is particularly pronounced in the U.S., where this organizational form has grown to cover over 50 percent of the population in some areas such as Massachusetts. Two-thirds of American workers with health insurance were enrolled in MCOs in 1999, compared to only 10 percent in 1990.

Managed care has evolved in the U.S. as a major means for restructuring the health system and how business is conducted within the system for several reasons. First, managed care seeks to improve

Figure 4.1
The Growth of HMOs in the U.S.

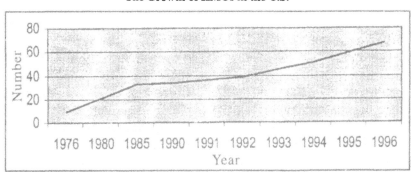

Source: National Center for Health Statistics, Health, United States, 1998 (Hyattsville, MD, 1998).

Figure 4.2
Enrollment in HMOs in the U.S.

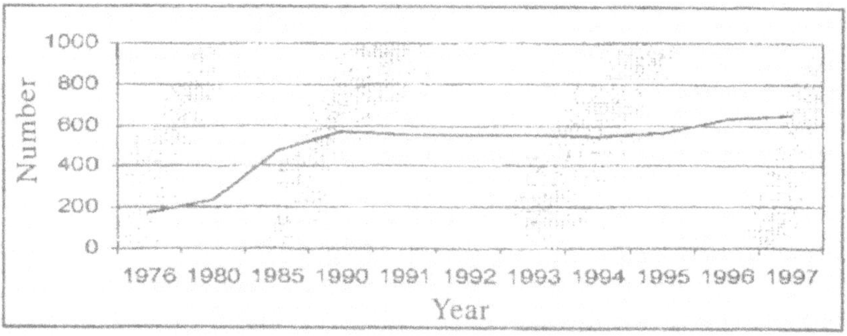

Source: National Center for Health Statistics, Health, United States, 1998.

the coordination of services and offers improved continuity of care as well as a continuum of care. Second, the need to control the costs of health care has precipitated the dramatic growth of managed care. Finally, it is attractive because it creates a system within the often confusing health care system of the U.S. to cover the services a population requires at a fixed cost.

What is Managed Care?

Managed care is the combining of a prepaid, capitated payment for health insurance with group medical practice as the means of delivery of services. Physician and hospital payments or reimbursement come from the subscribers' capitation payments. The physicians may be members of a prepaid group practice or a looser confederation of providers that have agreed to provide all necessary preventive, outpatient, and inpatient services for the agreed capitated fee. Hence managed care brings together the provision of health services with the financing of health services.

The basic benefits of managed care systems are affordability, effectiveness, and high quality. Since premiums are prepaid by a large population, managed care schemes spread risks while minimizing the financial exposure of subscribers. This risk pooling makes the premiums much more affordable. It is also an effective means of providing a wide range of health care services, from preventive to curative. Managed care also ensures quality of care by incorporating medical management and utilization review. Managed care schemes monitor the quality of care by providers, both physicians and hospitals, as well as the scheme's members' utilization of different providers. Managed care takes forms ranging from health maintenance organizations to preferred provider organizations, as discussed below.

Insurer and Provider Functions Combined

Health insurance has arisen because it protects people against the financial risks of health care if they suffer serious illness, for which the cost of treatment can be high and pose a financial hardship. Individuals find it worthwhile to contribute regularly to an insurance fund an amount equal to the average yearly costs of covered care for a group of people. By making regular small payments (premiums), individuals are protected against the risk of ever having to pay the full cost of a catastrophic illness. Insurance shares the burden of payment for illness among all the members of the scheme whether they be ill or healthy, poor or non-poor. Hence, the basic purpose of insurance is risk pooling. This type of indemnity insurance pays the cost of health services for each episode of illness for the conditions or services covered by the insurance. Under these arrangements, there are three distinct parties: the insured (or member), the provider of health services, and the insurer. The insurer receives money from the insured and provides money to providers, who in turn deliver services to the member.

Managed care is another form of health insurance in that it pools the risks of illness of a group of people. It is different from indemnity health insurance because it integrates the financing and delivery of care. However, rather than simply paying providers for the services delivered, the managed care organization employs physicians and may contract with or own the clinics and hospitals from which services are provided to its covered members. It not only finances care but also arranges or directly provides all medical care for the covered population. Members are not free to choose any provider but must choose from the managed care plan's providers or those with whom it has contracted. There is a network of providers, who are reimbursed by various combinations of capitation and fee-for-service payments. The providers may be staff or facilities of the plan, and they usually provide comprehensive benefits that include preventive services. There are limited cost-sharing charges, such as copayments at time of service to discourage unnecessary visits.

A managed care organization (MCO) shares some risks because it is responsible for providing a comprehensive range of services to its members. It is at risk for providing necessary care to its entire population within a fixed budget, upon which its premiums are based. To control costs, an MCO uses design of benefits, cost sharing, and provider payment mechanisms to influence utilization and ultimately costs, like traditional private indemnity insurance. Extensive medical management and utilization review are used to maintain quality standards among providers and appropriate utilization of services by both providers and the insured.

Because the insured individuals, or members, in a managed care plan must use only the providers within the plan or those under contract with the plan, an MCO has greater control over the providers and their behavior than a traditional health insurance agency. An MCO is thus able to control costs to a greater extent. Table 4.1 summarizes the important features of MCOs.

Table 4.1
Key Elements of Managed Care

Key Element	Characteristics
Financing and provision combined	Insurance and health care services are combined into a single product.
Principles of insurance	Program and benefit eligibility are established using insurance principles.
Comprehensive services	Coverage is provided for a broad range of health care services: preventive and curative, inpatient and outpatient.
Provider network	Services are generally available through a preselected network of providers, such as a group practice of physicians who are under contract to the sponsor.
Capitation payments	The program generally provides all necessary services for a predetermined, prepaid monthly premium.
Gatekeeper	The patient may be required to follow certain protocols to obtain care, such as seeing specialist physicians only when referred by the primary care provider.
Active management of care	The plan oversees the care and cost of treatment to members and uses processes to control costs and utilization, such as competitive bidding to buy drugs at the lowest cost or pre-admission reviews to ensure that each hospital stay is required.
Risk sharing	The providers and MCO each accept the financial risk that if covered members require more or costlier care than anticipated, they are liable for the financial shortfall.

Coordination of Provider, Financier, and Client Perspectives

Combining the financier and provider in a managed care plan requires the plan to assume the perspective of its members, since it is responsible for their complete care and requires their support to prevent unnecessary utilization of services. MCOs are therefore unique because they combine the perspectives of the three main actors: providers, insurers, and members. The rationale is that no single actor can determine the quality and cost of the services. A cooperative understanding between the three parties is necessary for a successful MCO.

Under traditional insurance, the insurer is concerned primarily with paying for services, not with ensuring the quality of those services. The provider is concerned primarily with providing high-quality care and is not concerned with the cost of covered services. The client wants unlimited high-quality health services with low premiums and is not concerned about the cost of the services covered by insurance. These conflicting objectives, along with a lack of coordinated effort, cause many of the problems associated with traditional indemnity health insurance.

MCOs require compromises, since it is not possible to achieve all of these objectives simultaneously. For example, it is not possible to have unlimited high-quality services and to reimburse providers at high rates while controlling costs and keeping premiums and copayments low for subscribers. An MCO structure, which integrates the financing and delivery of services, can be both cost effective and responsive to members= needs.

Elements of a Managed Care System

Five elements of managed care distinguish it from other forms of health insurance:

1. *Care arranged by the primary care physician.* The MCO plan seeks the lowest-level provider who is qualified to deliver appropriate services. Since primary care physicians can handle the majority of subscribers' care needs, these physicians serve as a gatekeeper handling entry into and referral within the system.

2. *Organized system and network of providers.* An MCO provides continuity of care for subscribers by using primary care physicians to manage the care received. Subscribers cannot refer themselves to specialists but must be referred by primary care physicians. Because primary care physicians provide most of

the care, the MCO often contracts with specialists only for necessary services rather than employing them. MCO plans may also utilize ancillary health personnel to provide services under the direction of a physician. These may include paramedics, physician assistants, nurse practitioners, or clinic officers.

3.   *Health promotion and maintenance.* Because the MCO is responsible for the total care of the covered population, preventive and promotive services are usually included in the benefit package because they improve health, reduce risk of disease, and thereby reduce the MCOs future financial obligations for treating preventable illnesses and conditions. This holds true only if there is an expected long-term relationship between the covered members and the MCO. The MCO also attempts to reduce or eliminate medically unnecessary tests and treatments and to focus upon the most cost-effective services.

4.   *Fixed budget financed by a predetermined premium.* The "insurance premium" under an MCO is a payment made in advance of the period of service, usually monthly or quarterly. The MCO can predict its cash flow because it knows the number of subscribers and the premium it charges.

5.   *Risk sharing.* By having a prepaid insurance premium and being responsible for total care, MCOs assume financial risk if expenditures for services exceed income from premiums. The MCO is operating on a fixed budget. It provides a package of benefits and bases its premiums on historical and expected utilization rates. If utilization is higher than expected, the MCO is at financial risk because expenses will be higher but revenues are fixed by the prepaid premiums. To help manage this risk, MCOs often contract with service providers to assume part of the financial risk of unexpected high utilization. This risk sharing can be accomplished by basing provider fees on a capitation basis or a fixed budget rather than on the number of services provided. Providers therefore have some incentive to keep costs within the budgeted amount by promoting preventive services, which will minimize the quantity of curative services the MCO will have to provide. Premiums for indemnity insurance are determined by actual utilization of individuals and groups in the prior period. If utilization goes up, premiums will increase or benefits be reduced or both, to balance the increased costs with the revenues.

MCO Payment Mechanisms

Payment mechanisms may encourage providers to increase prices for services and promote increased use or quantity of services. To share these risks with providers, MCOs often use payment mechanisms such as capitation or fixed budgets, which are closed-ended, instead of open-ended payment mechanisms such as fee-for-service payments, which are often used in indemnity health insurance plans. Table 4.2 illustrates some alternative payment mechanisms and their intended incentives:

- *Fee-for-service.* With a fee-for-service payment system, the provider establishes a charge for each service and either the patient or the insurance fund pays that amount to the provider without negotiation. In this situation there is no constraint on the price per service or the quantity of services provided.

- *Flat rate or payment per day (all-inclusive per diem).* A flat rate is a method of paying for inpatient hospital services based upon a daily rate for care provided. This rate is considered payment in full for services, regardless of the types of services provided to the patient or the costs of those services. The hospital tariff is an example of a payment per day.

- *Payment per case or admission.* Payment per case is similar to payment per day, except that the payment is fixed for each admission to the hospital regardless of the patient's diagnosis, the complexity of treatment, or the length of stay.

- *Capitation payment.* Capitation is a payment system that is calculated based on the number of members served by a specific physician or hospital. Hence total revenues are the fixed rate times the number of covered members. Revenues are not tied to utilization of services. The provider is paid a fixed amount per member per month regardless of how many patients are treated.

- *Budget or block payment.* The provider is paid a negotiated amount in return for providing an estimated volume of service. The payment is usually negotiated for a year and paid monthly. The hospital must provide statistics on service utilization by the group for whom the block payment is made.

- *Performance contract.* A performance contract is an agreement that specifies certain performance targets, such as immunization coverage or covered population. Insurance funds can use such agreements with providers, particularly hospitals, to encourage improvements in the quality and cost-effectiveness of health services.

The first three payment methods (fee-for-service, flat rate per day, and payment per case) are open-ended. The amount paid for services is determined by the price multiplied by the number of units of service. The health insurance fund bears the financial risk. For example, if the number of service units, and hence the total payments, is greater than anticipated, the fund is responsible for the additional cost. Open-ended systems create an incentive for providers to increase service utilization in order to increase revenues.

The next two payment methods (capitation and budget payment) are closed-ended. The amount paid by the fund is unrelated to the level of service utilization. The providers (usually hospitals) bear part of the financial risk. The hospital bears the additional cost if the

Table 4.2
Performance under Different Provider Payment Systems

Provider Payment System	Expected Utilization Changes	Expected Total Cost Changes	Cost Containment Incentives	Administrative Complexity
Fee-for-service	Increases utilization	Increases total costs	Weak	Complex
Flat rate	Increases utilization	Increases total costs	Average	Uncomplicated
Payment per case	—	Increases total costs	Average	Complex
Capitation payment	↓Decreases utilization	↓Decreases total costs	Strong	Uncomplicated
Fixed budget	↓Decreases utilization	↓Decreases total costs	Strong	Uncomplicated
Performance contract	↓Decreases utilization	↓Decreases total costs	Strong	Uncomplicated

cost of providing services to members is greater than the amount received from the fund or it benefits if the cost of providing services to covered members is less than the payments or premiums received from the MCO. These systems contain incentives for providers to seek the most cost-effective methods of providing the necessary services and reduce the cost of services. They may result in inadequate care, denial of necessary treatment, or other inappropriate measures to reduce costs. The fund must monitor service provision to ensure that quality of care is not being compromised.

Organizational Elements of Managed Care Organizations

Forms of Managed Care Organizations

There are four basic forms of MCOs. The first, the health maintenance organization (HMO), is well known. HMOs provide comprehensive services for their members for a fixed, prepaid fee. HMOs are organized health systems responsible for both financing and providing a broad range of comprehensive services to an enrolled population.

There are several models of HMOs, which are continually changing and expanding in an effort to remain competitive and attract subscribers. HMOs use a variety of cost-containment procedures to control the unnecessary use of health services. Primary care physicians treat patients and authorize and direct all other services provided to enrollees. Providers, both primary care physicians and specialists, may be employees of the HMO and be paid by salary, fee-for-service, or a capitation fee for each patient enrolled with them as their primary care provider. MCOs may tie the payment of providers to performance by including incentives for exceeding performance targets, such as bonuses, and disincentives for not meeting targets, such as withholding of payments. Table 4.3 illustrates typical financial arrangements between providers and MCOs.

As to facilities, the HMO may own their own hospitals or contract with hospitals for services for their members. Many have clinical guidelines that providers are expected to follow.

A second type of MCO is the preferred provider organization (PPO). PPOs are entities through which employer health benefit plans and health insurance carriers contract to purchase health care services from a selected group of participating providers. They are MCOs in which there are a limited number of health care providers—physicians and hospitals—who agree to provide services for enrollees at a negotiated fee-for-service rate that is less than their usual charge. PPOs provide a choice of health care providers for patients from a list of approved providers. Beneficiaries are often permitted to visit non-contracted physicians and hospitals, but only at added costs, such as higher deductibles or copayments.

The PPO model does not require patients to see a gatekeeper or primary care physician first. They are free to consult with specialists. Physician providers are allowed to maintain their office practices on a fee-for-service basis. They may be part of multiple PPOs as well as seeing patients that are not enrolled in MCOs. The PPOs attempt to manage costs by requiring pre-authorization of non-urgent hospital admissions, conducting utilization review of providers, often requiring a second opinion for surgery, and doing studies that compare the treatment provided by their physicians with that of physicians in other practice settings.

Table 4.3

Financial Arrangements between Providers and Managed Care Organizations

Financial Arrangement	Description
Discounted fee-for-service	A portion of each payment is withheld depending upon the performance of the provider. If the provider's performance relative to costs and quality has been maintained, the full payments are made and a bonus possibly paid.
Capitation	• Payment is made on a capitated basis for each enrollee selecting that provider. A bonus or withholding of a portion of the payment is possible depending upon the performance of each provider. • The primary care physician gives all or part of the total care to the member. • Specialists may be employed under special arrangements and paid for a percentage of their time or on a capitated or fee-for-service basis.
Salary	Providers are paid a salary regardless of how many patients they see or who are enrolled with them. There may be a withholding pending evaluation of performance for quality and patient satisfaction, as well as a bonus for exceeding targets.

A third form of MCO is the exclusive provider organization (EPO). An EPO is similar to a PPO except that beneficiaries can seek care only from the preferred providers. If members seek care from other providers, the cost of those services is not covered.

Finally, a point-of-service (POS) plan is a hybrid of an HMO and a PPO. Primary care physicians are employed or contracted with and paid on a capitation basis. These physicians act as gatekeepers, but members are permitted to go outside the network by assuming greater financial burdens through higher copayments, deductibles, or both. Usually the premiums of POS are higher than HMOs or PPOs since the enrollees are paying a higher premium in exchange for greater freedom of choice and flexibility in choosing providers who may not be part of the network. Financial risk is shared in that only partial payments are made to physicians in case utilization is higher than expected. At the end of the year, if usage by the population is greater than what the premium was based on, there is a pro rata cut in the payments to providers. If actual visits are equal to or fewer than expected, the balance due for full payments is made to providers.

Table 4.4 summarizes the impact of these various types of MCO on members and their freedom of choice in selecting the provider from whom they will receive care.

How Do MCOs Differ from Indemnity Health Insurance?

The usual form of indemnity insurance separates the financing and provision of health care. With indemnity insurance, the insurer's liability is determined by a fixed predetermined amount for a covered event. The member or employer pays a premium to the insurance company for the health services covered by the insurance policy. Sets of services vary in their level of comprehensiveness. Policies may exclude preexisting conditions, have maximum payment amounts, or simply not cover certain conditions. The member will have total free choice in selecting a provider, who submits bills to the insurance company on a fee-for-service basis. Members are responsible for coordinating their own care.

By contrast, MCOs cover a comprehensive set of services, their premium is an all-encompassing monthly premium, and the providers are either part of the MCO or have negotiated contracts with the MCO to provide services, with payment on a capitation basis or at a discounted price.

Table 4.4
Impact of the Type of Managed Care Organizations on the Members

Type of MCO	Impact on Members
HMO	No freedom of choice of provider. Access to specialists is through the principal care provider or gatekeeper.
Preferred provider organization	There is no gatekeeper, so the member has freedom of choice to opt out of the network of providers but at the cost of paying higher out-of-pocket payments.
Exclusive provider organization	There is no freedom of choice in that care provided outside the network of providers is not covered. So while there is no gatekeeper, the member has freedom of choice to opt out only if he or she is willing to assume total financial responsibility. Services outside the network are not covered.
Point of service	There is a gatekeeper but members have the freedom to opt out of the network of providers by assuming higher out-of-pocket payments.

Managed Care Competition

MCOs have the common goal of reducing health expenditure while maintaining quality of care. This is supposed to be achieved in part through competition in quality and cost, meaning that consumers must be informed and involved in choosing their health insurance plan. In advanced stages of MCO development, as in the U.S., competition between MCOs can have a positive impact on the cost and quality of health services. When MCOs compete, their success in attracting new members is based on offering good-quality, accessible services at an affordable price. The most effective competitors excel in balancing these somewhat contradictory objectives. Competition between MCOs produces much less inflation of health costs than does competition between indemnity health insurance plans. Indemnity health insurance plans have traditionally had limited, if any, cost containment provisions; they usually contain incentives for providers to increase utilization in order to maximize fee income.

However, the emphasis on cost containment has been so great in some instances that some people believe that MCOs have reduced quality and put covered members at risk by discharging inpatients from hospitals sooner than is medically appropriate. The result has been government interventions, such as laws to require MCOs to allow women to stay in the hospital up to two days after delivery rather than forcing same-day delivery discharges.

Managed Care in the U.S.

A Brief History of Managed Care Organizations in the U.S.

Prior to the 1960s, there were few pioneers in managed care. A few early MCOs include the Community Hospital Association of Elk City, Oklahoma (1929), Ross Loos Clinic in Los Angeles (1929), the Group Health Cooperative of Puget Sound (1935), Kaiser Foundation Health Plan in California (1942), and the Health Insurance Plan of New York (1946). These plans grew out of special needs and circumstances of the moment. For example, the Kaiser Foundation Health Plan developed from the need to establish a health insurance plan for many workers in the shipyards in California during World War II. The prepaid group practice model was adopted. It was not until the 1970s that MCOs became prominent. The term health maintenance organization was introduced in 1971 to refer to a group of independent insurance plans that combined capitated prepayments with group practice provision of services. The federal government financially supported their development with the Health Maintenance Organization Act of 1973. There were several reasons for this rise in managed care.

The rapid inflation of the cost of medical care in the U.S. in the 1960s and 1970s created a demand for health insurance products that would provide incentives to inhibit cost inflation. The environment of the early 1970s was ripe for change. Cost inflation resulted in wage and price controls, the passage of certificate of need legislation, the establishment of rate-setting commissions in many states to regulate price increases by providers, and the establishment of professional standards review organizations for Medicare. Secondly, there was a shifting of the role of the physician in U.S. society. With the rise of the women's movement, patients started to demand a greater say in their care. This change had an impact on the male-dominated area of medical care. Additionally, there was evidence that the cost and quality of care were not correlated. Hence, there was a desire to obtain cost-effective care, and MCOs were seen as a means for achieving this.

As a result, the HMO Act of 1973 was passed. The government sought to facilitate the development of prepaid health schemes by providing subsidies for the development of HMOs. They also mandated that employers begin offering HMOs as an option for employees for their health insurance.

Managed Care in the Public Sector

There are two large public health insurance programs in the U.S., Medicare for the elderly and disabled and Medicaid for the poor. Before recent reforms, both public programs provided their covered populations with insurance similar to the traditional indemnity insurance available in the private sector. Rapid escalation of the costs of these programs inspired reform of provider payment mechanisms and, more recently, the incorporation of MCOs as an option for beneficiaries.

Medicare was introduced in 1965 to reduce financial barriers to health care services for the elderly population in the U.S. This social insurance program was introduced in response to the fact that most elderly people had relatively low incomes and could not afford to pay for care, and private insurance companies were reluctant to sell them health insurance policies. Medicare is a federally funded and administered system, in contrast to Medicaid, the U.S. health insurance program for the poor, which is state administered and funded by a combination of state and federal funds. Elderly people who are also poor receive health insurance from Medicare and additional coverage to fund copayments, prescription drugs, and long-term care from Medicaid. Together, Medicare and Medicaid financed $351 billion in health care services in 1996, which represents more than one-third of total U.S. spending on health.

Growth of managed care in U.S. public health insurance. The number of people covered by Medicaid grew from 23 million in 1975 to 41 million in 1996. Of the 41 million people covered by Medicaid in 1996, 4.7 million or 13 percent were enrolled in managed care organizations (see Figure 4.3). Medicare enrollment grew from 25.7 million in 1976 to 41 million in 1996. In 1996, 9.7 percent of Medicare enrollees were in managed care plans, a more than 300 percent increase since 1985 (see Figure 4.4).

Figure 4.3
The Growth of Medicaid

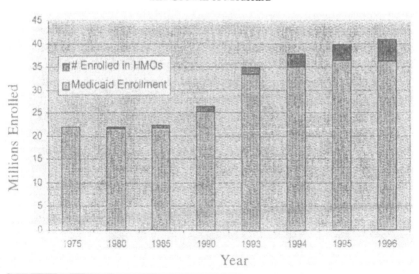

Source: National Center for Health Statistics, Health, United States, 1998 (Hyattsville, MD, 1998).

Figure 4.4
The Growth of Medicare

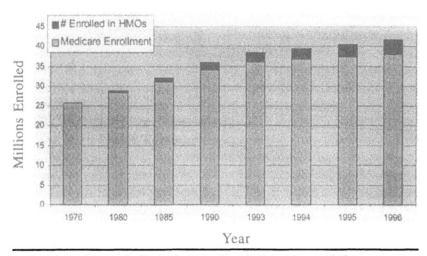

Source: National Center for Health Statistics, Health, United States, 1998.

Managed care for the elderly and poor. Since 1985, health maintenance organizations (HMOs) have been allowed to contract with the government to assume the financial risk of providing at least the full package of Medicare benefits to those who enroll.2 Medicare beneficiaries have a choice between traditional fee-for-service indemnity insurance with copayments and deductibles or HMOs that are qualified by the Health Care Financing Administration, the public entity that manages the Medicare program, to provide Medicare recipients with health care services. Qualified HMOs are required to take any Medicare participant who chooses to enroll. HMOs are paid a monthly premium, the adjusted average per capita cost (AAPCC), which is equivalent to 95 percent of the average amount Medicare would have paid for a beneficiary of similar age and the same gender in that geographic area. Criticism of this method arose from findings suggesting that healthier-than-average beneficiaries choose HMOs.3 These beneficiaries would have cost Medicare less than the average of those with similar profiles had they remained in the traditional fee-for-service Medicare program. The result could be that paying HMOs based on AAPCC rates could end up costing the Medicare program more than the traditional program. Work is under way to improve the calculation of the Medicare risk premiums.

Medicaid is a state-managed social insurance system, funded with a combination of state and federal funds. The federal government determines a basic package of benefits that must be provided to the population of a state that meets at least minimal federal requirements. States are free to both increase the package of benefits they cover and increase the level of income over the federally determined poverty line they will cover. Many states have moved toward a Medicaid system that has eliminated traditional indemnity insurance as an option and gives recipients a choice among competing MCOs. Premiums are established differently in different states but competitive bidding is being implemented in many places.

Evidence of the impact of MCOs on Medicare and Medicaid. Since HMOs assume the full risk of providing the complete Medicare or Medicaid package of benefits for a predetermined monthly premium, they face incentives to increase efficiency and to control costs. There is concern that these incentives will cause HMOs to provide too little care and that quality will suffer. The media in the U.S. have focused largely on isolated negative events and paid less attention to assessing the broader picture of managed care. Data are not consistent, which makes it difficult for researchers to compare quality and performance, and for policymakers and consumers to choose plans based on reliable information. Miller and Luft[4] looked at 68 studies of managed care performance that compared quality in HMOs to quality in fee-for-service health plans. The results showed that some HMOs provide better quality and others worse. There was some consistency in that HMOs were reported to provide lower-quality care to the chronically ill elderly, causing the researchers to recommend future studies that focus on different population groups. In addition, the degree of HMO market penetration[5] affects both market-wide prices and clinical practices for all patients in a region. Some cost-cutting measures, such as reducing expensive diagnostic tests, are easy to implement. However, as HMO market penetration increases, a more comprehensive re-engineering of clinical practices could evolve, with the potential to improve quality of care as well as lower costs.

The Impact of Managed Care

To provide high-quality health services while containing costs, MCOs promote efficiency among providers, pay only for treatments and medicines that are proven to be effective for a given condition, and avoid paying for services or procedures whose value is unknown or that have proven to be less than cost effective. The specific ways in which MCOs have affected the U.S. health care industry are discussed below.

Costs of Medical Care

Managed care has reduced the cost of services. HMOs have been found to provide comparable coverage and services at costs that were 14.7 percent less than traditional indemnity insurance, while PPOs has 6.1 percent lower costs than traditional indemnity insurance. The Academy for International Health Studies has asserted that HMOs are 18 percent more efficient than indemnity health insurance plans without any adverse effect on quality of care.[6] The government has encouraged, but not mandated, people covered under Medicare to enroll in MCOs to control the rise of costs without compromising quality of care or access to services. MCOs manage medical costs in a variety of ways, as shown in Tables 4.2 and 4.3. For example, providers share financial risk through capitation, which creates the incentive to reduce both unit costs and the quantity of services used. The resulting impact of MCOs in the U.S. health systems has been:

- reduction in overall spending growth on health care by reducing the number of hospitals and changing how providers were paid;

- increased use of ambulatory or outpatient care for many conditions that were previously treated on an inpatient basis;

- major organizational changes in how health care is delivered, from many providers in solo practice or small group practices of two to four physicians to most physicians belonging to one or more networks of physicians of varying degrees of formality.

Practice of Medicine

The practice of medicine has changed under the influence of managed care. The role of the physician has shifted from being simply the agent of the patient, with the patient being the provider's sole focus of concern in making choices of treatment and care. The new role that has developed for physicians in MCOs is the responsibility to balance the needs of the individual patient with the goals of the larger system. For example, as medical technology has advanced, the system has been able to improve quality while reducing costs by safely performing many uncomplicated, minor surgical procedures, which had previously been done exclusively on an inpatient basis, on an outpatient basis.

The advent of MCOs has also resulted in the practice patterns of physicians being examined much more closely. Previously a physician's practice patterns may have only been noticed when they were at the extremes beyond the usual norms of practice. With managed care there is increased feedback to physicians about their clinical performance. They also receive much more information on the norms of practice for particular procedures, so there is a much stronger push for moving toward the mean and much less variation in practice norms. Part of this is accomplished through treatment algorithms and active management of drug formularies for physicians. There is a much more educational support for physicians, in addition to the advantages they receive from practicing in groups rather than as individual practitioners.

Quality of Care

The movement of physicians' treatment patterns toward the norm due to education, closer interaction with colleagues, and greater oversight of their practice patterns has improved quality, particularly for common health problems. However, there are potential risks to quality in MCOs as well as possibilities of quality improvement. Quality may be at risk when the need for approval from the primary care physician-gatekeeper causes delays in treatment. Due to the referrals required, there is also the possibility of care being inappropriately denied. Although much of the recent criticism of MCOs focuses on the denial of care, there is evidence that the number of denied treatments is small: less than 1 percent of surgical procedures recommended are denied and less than 3 percent of physician-recommended treatments are denied.[7] There is also the possibility of care being delivered at the wrong level because of the physician-gatekeeper and the emphasis on decreasing hospitalization. MCOs address quality by developing standard diagnostic and treatment protocols or guidelines that physicians must use for common conditions. In addition, MCOs have rigorous peer review to compare clinical outcomes and evaluate clinical treatments in an attempt to ensure the maintenance of a high standard of quality of care.

In efforts to ensure the quality of MCOs, the National Committee for Quality Assurance (NCQA) was formed in 1979. It became independent from the national MCO association in 1990 and in 1991 started to accredit MCOs. As part of this process, it began to release information on accreditation status to the public in 1994 and released refined quality indicator instruments in 1996 in the form of "report cards." The purposes of NCQA are to (1) provide accreditation of MCOs by overseeing, measuring, and assessing the performance of MCOs, (2) provide information on the quality of care provided by MCOs to the public, and (3) promote improvements in the quality of care provided by MCOs. The NCQA believes that true competition requires public information on the quality of MCOs and that this information will provide incentives for quality improvements for those MCOs not performing as well. The accreditation process of NCQA covers six areas with their relative weighting indicated below:

- Quality improvement (35%)

- Physician credentials (25%)

- Members' rights and responsibilities (10%)

- Utilization management (10%)

- Medical records (10%)

- Preventive health services (10%)

Member Satisfaction

In general, enrollees are satisfied with the care and treatment they receive from their MCOs. A survey of Medicare enrollees in MCOs found them satisfied but less so than enrollees in Medicare fee-for-service plans that had unlimited options.[8] Private-sector employers offering MCOs as an insurance option to their employees are increasingly requiring that they be accredited by the NCQA to ensure that quality is maintained. Many of these employers actually use quality of care data in making choices about which MCOs to offer their employees. Yet there is a concern that in the effort to contain costs, quality of care may suffer for various reasons: patients may wait longer for appointments, fewer referrals will be made to specialists and for diagnostic tests, and needed care will not be provided. Thus quality of care has become a significant concern for those enrolled in MCOs.

Organization of the Health Care System

Managed care has radically changed the roles of purchasers, insurers, the insured, physicians, and hospitals. It has shifted the predominant means of charging for services from fee-for-service payment to capitated basis. It has also resulted in the development of many new products or arrangements among the insured members, providers, and financiers or insurers. The result has been new forms of MCOs as well as differing means for managing those providers to ensure the provision of high-quality care in a cost-effective manner. It success is evidenced by the migration of members from indemnity health insurance forms to MCOs as the predominant means by which those who are insured are covered for health services that they need.

The Future of Managed Care in the U.S.

Managed care has sought to improve quality through education, improved preventive care, close monitoring of physicians, special programs to manage chronic conditions, and treatment and drug protocols for various conditions. MCOs have demonstrated that costs can be controlled through managing the use of the health care system and changing incentives that alter behavior. The initial years of managed care brought large gains in cost control as length of stay in hospitals fell and the number of diagnostic tests per enrollee was reduced. Over time, however, efficiency gains will come from more fundamental restructuring of the way care is organized and delivered.

The health care marketplace and managed care organizations will continue to evolve in the U.S. due to concerns about maximizing quality while controlling costs. Cost control pressure from employers, who are the major purchasers of health care, will drive health plans to introduce more innovations in organization and delivery that control costs. In some regions employers are joining coalitions of employers who negotiate with health plans as a group and insist on quality as well as low costs. This move toward getting value for money and an emphasis on performance are expected to encourage health plans to focus more on quality of care.

Despite these positive achievements of controlling costs and enhancing quality for the U.S. health system as a result of the expansion of MCOs, there has been increasing signs of public discontent with this form of health care delivery. While the evidence indicates that quality of care appears to be good in managed care plans, coverage in the media has undermined public confidence in MCO institutions. In response, President Clinton has appointed a commission to study quality of care and recommend ways to improve measurement of quality and accountability to consumers. There has also been attempts to legislate additional rights for patients to be able to seek redress for grievances against MCOs in the legal system's courts. Much of the discontent has arisen from restrictions on the free choice of provider for members of MCOs as well as patients' perceptions of quality deficiencies in the care provided by MCOs. Though the evidence indicates that MCOs have improved not decreased quality, the public believe that quality has suffered in the form of fewer services due to the emphasis MCOs place on controlling costs. MCOS will face increasing pressures to respond to consumer preferences of wanting greater freedom of choice in selection of their individual provider. The result will be the creation of additional variations of the MCO structure to allow greater freedom for enrollees to visit their provider of choice. However, this pressure creates a tension in the objectives of MCOs because as freedom of choice can be increased only at the expense of dilution of cost control gains. The challenge for MCOs and the U.S. health system for the future will be to regain public confidence and be able to demonstrate the positive effect of MCOs on quality, while limiting the freedom of choice of providers enough to allow for maintaining control of health care costs.

The Future of Managed Care in Other Countries

Countries throughout the world, and at all levels of development, are struggling to find ways to deliver high-quality health care services with limited budgets. Aspects of managed care have potential applications in social insurance systems and private systems around the world. Managed health care has strong potential applications in the high-cost industrialized countries of Western Europe[9] and Japan and newly industrialized countries such as Korea. Managed health care also has potential applications in transitional economies such as those of Russia, the NIS, Eastern Europe, and Mongolia, for example, where loosely defined and poorly managed health insurance programs are springing up to compensate for declining government payments to the health sector. In many of these countries, government-supported group practice or polyclinic models form potential building blocks for effective managed care systems. Health reforms in Latin America are moving toward competition among health plans that accepted capitated payments to provide a defined benefits package to the population. Tools of managed care are currently being implemented and more fundamental changes in the organization and delivery of health services can be expected.

Notes

1. McGreevey, W. P., Social Security in Latin America: Options for the World Bank, World Bank Discussion Paper No. 110 (The World Bank, November 1990); Lewis, J. presentation on managed care at the Second International Health Economists Association meeting in Rotterdam, June 1999.
2. Many Medicare HMOs include more benefits than required under Medicare, such as coverage for prescription drugs and reduced copayments.
3. Brown, R. et al., "Do Health Maintenance Organizations Work for Medicare?" Health Care Financing Review 15 (Fall 1993):7-23.
4. Miller, R. H. and Luft, H. S. "Does Managed Care Lead to Better or Worse Quality of Care?" Health Affairs 16 (Sept.-Oct. 1997):7-25.
5. HMO market penetration is defined as the percentage of the population of a region that is enrolled in an HMO. Since HMOs contract with hospitals and doctors that also serve people in fee-for-service plans, a higher degree of HMO market penetration would be expected to change the clinical practices of health providers for all people, regardless of health plan.
6. Lewis, presentation at the Second International Health Economics Association Conference, 1999.
7. Ibid.
8. Adler, G. S. "Medicare Beneficiaries Rate their Medical Care—New Data from MCBS," Health Care Financing Review 16 (1995):175.
9. European Health Care Trends: Towards Managed Care in Europe (Coopers & Lybrand Europe, 1995).

References

Adler, G. S. "Medicare Beneficiaries Rate their Medical Care—New Data from MCBS." Health Care Financing Review 16 (1995):175.
Brown, R., et al. "Do Health Maintenance Organizations Work for Medicare?" Health Care Financing Review 15 (Fall 1993):7-23.

Devers, K. J. "The Challenges of Implementing Market-Based Reform for Public Clients." In Competitive Managed Care. San Francisco: Jossey-Bass Publishers. 1997, pp. 259-96.

Eichler, R. "Financing Health Care for the Elderly in Competitive Health Plan Markets: Experiences from the United States and the Netherlands and Proposals for Reform." Unpublished manuscript. March 1999.

Enthoven, A. C. "Consumer Choice Health Plan: A National Health Insurance Proposal Based on Regulated Competition in the Private Sector." New England Journal of Medicine 298 (1978):709-20.

European Health Care Trends: Towards Managed Care in Europe. Coopers & Lybrand Europe, 1995.

Health Care Financing Administration. Health Care Financing Review: Medicare and Medicaid Statistical Supplement. 1998.

Lewis, J. Presentation on managed care at the Second International Health Economics Association meeting. Rotterdam, The Netherlands, June 1999.

McGreevey, W. P. Social Security in Latin America: Options for the World Bank. World Bank Discussion Paper No. 110. The World Bank, November 1990.

Miller, R. H. and Harold S. Luft. "Does Managed Care Lead to Better or Worse Quality of Care?" Health Affairs 16 (Sept.-Oct. 1997):7-25.

Raffel, M., ed. Health Care and Reform in Industrialized Countries. University Park, PA: Pennsylvania State University Press, 1997.

Robinson, J. C. "The Future of Managed Care." Health Affairs 18 (March-Apr. 1999):7-24.

5

China: Innovations in Health Care Financing—Mixing Individual and Collective Responsibility

A. Hu

After a half century's execution, China's old urban health insurance regime will be replaced by a Basic Health Insurance System for Urban Working People (BHISFUWP), and a new era in health insurance development will be opened when the market-oriented economy enters the twenty-first century.[1]

The new health protection mechanism is in response to the need for restructuring the old system, a point raised as early as the 1980s following economic reform. The old system, comprising one scheme for state-owned enterprise (SOE) and collective-owned enterprise (COE) workers and another for government employees, was actually entirely financed and run by individual employers, so it cannot continue to assume the same role in China's new market-led economy. There are two major defects in the old system: frequent failure to secure benefit payments in full and in time due to financial difficulties suffered by some individual employers, and the exclusion of non-public-sector workers and the self-employed, who now constitute about one-third of the urban labor force and continue to grow while the public sector is shrinking.

Prior to the announcement of the decree, a number of pilot programs had already been conducted in numerous localities over the last decade in an attempt to come up with a blueprint of a feasible and suitable health insurance model for the country. However, the government could not make a final decision due to the delicate and complex nature of the reform and anticipated difficulties in its implementation. It was only in early 1998 when a new Cabinet of the State Council was formed and approved by the People's Assembly and Mr. Zhu Rong Ji took office as the Prime Minister that the government finally decided to move forward in regard to health insurance restructuring to accommodate the accelerated economic reform, together with national campaigns on securing retirement and unemployment benefit payments.

Such a determination was not less weakened by a series of economic and natural disasters in 1998, notably the Asian financial crisis and the dramatic floods which affected 200 million inhabitants.[2] By contrast, it was further strengthened by the increasing need for an appropriate health care insurance system as a result of the crisis. This may partially explain why the timetable for the establishment of the BHISFUWP has become so urgent.

Based on the need for reform, lengthy studies, piloting experiences, and largely influenced by the newly established old-age insurance system with two components, the national campaign for setting up the BHISFUWP in the country in line with the decree is now officially launched.

Having had a brief glance at the background of China's health protection mechanism, it is now useful to look into the very details of this newly created model in the following sections: principal provisions, main features, preliminary analysis, and conclusions.

Principal Provisions Stipulated by Decree No. 44

Personal Coverage

All urban-based establishments—including public and private, national and international, profit-making and non-profit-making—and their employees, retirees and layoffs are obliged to participate in the BHISFUWP. The possible inclusion of other categories, such as workers in township/village enterprises (TVEs), urban self-employed and their employees, is up to the provincial, municipal and autonomous regional governments to determine. It is thus estimated that 13 percent of the total population in China[3] (excluding the self-employed and TVE workers), equivalent to approximately 162 million persons, would fall into the category of compulsory coverage.

Two-tier Structure and Benefit Provision

Stipulated benefits, comprising only medical care while leaving sick pay still in the hands of the employers, are separately payable under the two components of the BHISFUWP: an individual medical account (IMA) for each insured person based on self-reliance principles and a collective health insurance pooling fund (HIPF) based on social insurance principles. Annual health spending of an insured person should be firstly charged against his/her personal IMA, provided the overall amount does not exceed 10 percent of the regional average annual salary. If exceeded, it is the responsibility of the HIPF to pay the rest of the bills up to an amount equal to 400 percent of the regional average annual salary. For any expenditures higher than that, the responsibility is then passed either to a state-financed complementary scheme in the case of civil servants or to an enterprise/industry-based voluntary scheme, if any.

As with the somewhat loose provisions on coverage, detailed regulations on the benefit package and the exact division drawn between the two tiers, etc., are to be decided by the local authorities according to each situation.

Contributions and Financing

Both employers' and employees' contributions are now required: 6 percent of a contributory payroll—without imposing a ceiling on the income—from employers and 2 percent from workers. These resources are destined only for financing prescribed benefits.

Due to the two-tier structure of the system, generated revenues are split into two parts as well: for an individual IMA, its income comes from contributions paid by the insured, which is equal to 2 percent of his/her salary, plus some credit derived from employers' contributions. It is not entirely clear at this stage whether the second resource is linked with contributions made by the individual employer or by all employers. However, the aggregate percentage of such redistributable employers' contributions could be up to 30 percent. The precise extent and the method of redistribution are again up to the local authorities to determine. But it is required to be in conformity with the defined scope of the first tier in the region and to be distributed by age group. With regard to the HIPF, the rest of the employers' contributions, equivalent to approximately 4.2 percent of the payroll, are earmarked for it.

The decree further stipulates that no fund transfer between the two tiers and between different IMAs is permitted, but unspent allocations under the same IMA owner's name can be carried over to the following budgeting year and the balance in a deceased member's IMA can be inherited by the designated heir(s).

Apart from employers' and workers' contributions, the government also contributes to the system both in the form of tax exemptions and in the form of subsidies for financing the entire running costs of the BHISFUWP, as well as for financing complementary health insurance schemes for civil servants.

Special Provisions

Certain favorable measures are envisaged for the following five categories:

- *civil servants*—join the BHISFUWP, but compensated by state-financed supplementary schemes;

- *retirees*—exempted from paying individual contributions, but with higher allocations to their IMAs and lower co-payment rates;

- *laid-off workers*—exempted from paying contributions, which, including both employer's and employee's, are made by re-employment service centers, calculated on a basis of 60 percent of the average regional annual wage in the preceding year (assuming the unemployed are treated equally);

- *workers*—possibly complemented by the establishment of enterprise-based supplementary programs financed by up to 4 percent of the payroll before taxation;

- *retired senior government officers, ex-revolutionaries, war veterans and injured soldiers*—exempted from participating in the BHISFUWP, but with continuing privileged entitlement to special provisions financed by the government.

Management and Supervision

As in other social security schemes in the country, the responsibility for developing and monitoring the national policy and legislation on health insurance and guiding and supervising the administration of the BHISFUWP falls under the competence of the Ministry of Labour and Social Security (MOLSS) in consultation with other government departments concerned, particularly with Ministries of Public Health and Finance and the government Auditing Agency. Consultation with social partners is not stipulated in the decree, but it may take place from time to time. As it is actually organized and operated in each region, the decree leaves considerably large scope on policy to local governments to enable them to adapt the new system to their own situation. Therefore, the duty of health insurance policymaking is shared between the central and local governments and is somewhat decentralized.

The decree makes it clear that schemes are to be organized and divided by geographical regions at prefecture level and above; parallel industrial or occupational schemes are not permitted. They should be administered by health insurance institutions instead of employers themselves. A supervising organ, comprising representatives from responsible government departments, employers' and employees' organizations, medical providers and external experts, is to be set up at each administrative level to monitor and oversee the performance of the funds.

To facilitate the smooth implementation of the system, two concrete measures are foreseen to be taken immediately. First, a national guideline is to be formulated jointly by line ministries to guide and standardize principal provisions, such as the scope and criteria of basic benefits, lists of reimbursable medicaments, diseases covered, qualifications for selected medical providers (hospitals and other institutions) and pharmaceuticals. Based on that, local authorities lay down regional standards and application measures. Secondly, the funds have to be strictly deposited into special fiscal accounts in a designated bank. This means that no expenses other than prescribed health-related costs can be charged against balances in these accounts; and the use of these accounts, including crediting and debiting, is put under the close supervision of the Inland Revenue and other related government departments to prevent and minimize any possible fund abuse.

Reform in the Public Health Sector

As the public health sector is the main medical provider in the country, reform is also under way in this sector to accommodate changes required by the establishment of the BHISFUWP. It currently concentrates on four aspects of reform:

- separate accounting and management of medical services and pharmaceutical sales and introduce a competitive mechanism to bring health providers' prices down;

- adjust the health price structure, which has been distorted on the one hand by higher prices on drugs and high-tech tests and on the other hand by lower-than-cost prices on medical services with professional inputs;

- strengthen the internal management of hospitals, pharmaceutical providers and other related institutions with the view to regulating the conduct of medical personnel, increase productivity and lower costs;

- reinforce in-service training and promote the quality of professional personnel, optimize the structure of medical institutions and resources across the country, and develop community-based medical utilities and services.

Outstanding Features of the New Chinese Model

By comparing the new system with the previous one, critics in China underline four characteristics of the BHISFUWP which actually reflect the objectives and main principles of the new health insurance system.

Low Benefit Level

Just prior to this important reform, the overall annual expenditure on health insurance accounted for Yuan 77,370 million in 1997, rising 28 times in a twenty-year period—or 19 percent annually—whilst the average annual increase in GDP was only 11 percent during the same period.[5] The government estimates such a growth rate cannot be supported in the long term and believes this constituted one of the main reasons for the failure of the old system.

Learning from these experiences, and taking into account the rapidly ageing population, the limited health resources available on the supply side and the political commitment for expanding coverage, policymakers insist that the benefit level should be kept within the contributors' capacity and consistent as much as possible with the pace of economic development in order to ensure that the whole system is economically sustainable in the long term and does not impede on the prosperity of the economy. As both the level of the economy and the financing capacity of the contributors are estimated to be still low in the medium term, it has been decided to formulate moderate benefit provisions which are further constrained and limited by the IMA's functioning, copayment requirement, insurable benefit ceiling, lists of insurable medicines, technical diagnostic tests and medical services, the limited number of contracted providers, etc. So, comparatively, the benefit level under the new system is inferior to that under the previous two-type schemes, especially under the scheme for civil servants. But it is thought that the general protection level is promoted, thanks to extended personal coverage.

Universal Personal Coverage

Universal coverage used to be achieved for the urban working population prior to the commencement of economic reform in 1978, when the urban residents accounted for only up to 8 percent of the total population[6] and urban workers were mainly concentrated in the state and collective sectors.

After half a century of industrialization and urbanization, especially since economic reform, coverage under the old system has shrunk considerably; about half the urban inhabitants, equal to 15 percent of the whole population,[7] were uninsured in the 1990s. This is because the old health insurance system failed to adapt to the market-led economy and the changed labor market. First, the urban economy no longer simply consists of SOEs and COEs, but it also includes joint-owned enterprises, share holdings, cooperatives, joint ventures, foreign companies, overseas Chinese (Hong Kong, Macau and Taiwan funded), private firms and self-employed persons, etc. With the rapid growth of the non-SOE/COE sector, its workforce amounted to 29 percent of overall urban employment in 1996,[8] and it is estimated that it will rise to more than one-third in 1999, while the overall number and size of urban residents have been growing more than three times over the last two decades, amounting to 379 million and 30.4 percent of the population of 12.5 billion in 1998, respectively.[9] This is illustrated in Table 5.1. Second, employer liability-run schemes prove to be too fragile in a market-oriented economy; many insured workers do not receive promised benefits due to financial difficulties facing their employers.

Table 5.1
Number of Employed Persons in Urban Areas by Ownerships
(year end)
(10,000 persons)

	1952	1978	1985	1990	1995	1996
Total	2486	9514	12808	16616	19093	19815
SOE	1580	7451	8990	10346	11261	11244
COE	23	2048	3324	3549	3147	3016
Joint owned			38	96	53	49
Share holding					317	363
Foreign funded			6	62	241	275
Hongkong, Macau & Taiwan funded				4	272	265
Other ownership				2	11	9
Private				57	485	620
Self-employed	883	15	450	614	1560	1709

Source: State Statistical Bureau: *China Statistical Yearbook*, China Statistical Publishing House, 1997.

The new system is aimed at re-achieving universal coverage in terms of the urban labor force. The first step is to include the whole range of workers of the formal sector, irrespective of their status in ownership, employment and occupation. Inclusion of the self-employed and workers in TVEs is also possible, but not compulsory at the national level in the initial phase.

Here TVEs are an interesting Chinese phenomenon because they link the urban and the rural, the primary, secondary and tertiary industries, and self-employed farmers and wage-earners. Before 1978, they were much less developed, with only 28 million workers and limited to the primary industry. Now they provide employment to 130 million people, which is about 35 percent of the total number of workers in the non-primary industry.[10] However, due to their origin, they are still officially considered as part of the rural rather than urban labor force. Future extension to other urban groups, either by incorporating existing special programs or by setting up separate schemes or by direct expansion, will be under consideration in due course.

Contributions by Both Employers and Employees

This is the first time in the history of health insurance development in the country for an insured person to make a direct contribution to the funds along with the employers' contribution. Actually, it is not entirely new to workers, as the new old-age insurance has already introduced this mechanism.

Technically, the shifting of the mechanism will not cause any substantial changes to the overall amount of collected contributions, nor to take-home income at the initial stage, because the gross salary of the insured is proportionally increased. But it will rise when the contributory revenue of the insured subsequently grows.

The aim of introducing employees' contributions is to change the traditional concept that it is the duty of enterprises and the government to provide benefits and that the workers are only beneficiaries. By making workers into contributors as well, rising costs would also become their concern; thus, they would be keen to contain cost rises, to promote compliance and to accept self-control impositions as well.

Combination of the IMAs and the HIPF

This is the most notable characteristic of the new system, which distinguishes it from both its own past mechanism and other health care mechanisms in the world, because it combines a component based on traditional social insurance principles and a component based on provident fund principles into one mechanism. Because of this type of combination, it may provoke worldwide concern and debate on the appropriateness of the new system.

No matter how critics view this innovation, the inventors believe it is feasible and acceptable in the Chinese culture, where people have every intention to make savings (see Table 5.2) and this would probably apply to the IMAs. Thus, costs would be self-contained, and resources allocated to the tier of the IMAs would be economically used. In the first place, again it is estimated that, thanks to the existing high balance of family savings, it will not cause severe financial hardship for the insured individuals in case financing gaps occur between the current year's allocation and expenditure in certain IMAs. Also, the inclusion of an HIPF component builds up a "safety net" to secure basic protection for all insured people. Therefore, the government is convinced that with this two-tier portfolio, one based on the self-support principle and the other on solidarity, the new model can effectively protect the population at minimum cost.

Challenges and Difficulties Facing the Newly Innovated System

After a decade of consideration, research and experimentation, the orientation, principles and structure of the new health insurance system have been clarified and determined in China. This is being followed up by concrete designing and operating of regional schemes. Obviously, it is too early to assess the new system thoroughly. Nevertheless, the government should be aware of its potential weaknesses, various implications and possible ideas for improvement. Some preliminary analyses are highlighted below:

Personal Coverage: Is It Effective?

For the new health insurance system to effectively protect the targeted 162 million persons at once at the initial stage, there are considerable difficulties to be confronted. In particular, four issues have to be addressed:

• *The lack of necessary expertise and administrative infrastructures.* This is one consequence of the old system run by individual employers. Despite the fact that the BHISFUWP can somewhat benefit from previous experimenting experiences and receive support from certain common social insurance services such as data base and contribution collection, institution building still requires time and resources. The decree stipulates that all operational-related expenses are met by general revenues of local governments at the same administrative level. Thus, whether all responsible local authorities are financially able to make intensive

Table 5.2
Aggregate and Per Capita Balance of Savings Deposits
(year end)

	1978	1980	1985	1990	1995	1996
Outstanding amount (Yuan 100 million)	210.6	399.5	1622.6	7034.2	29662.3	38520.8
Per capita balance (Yuan)	21.88	40.47	153.29	615.24	2448.96	3163.8

Source: State Statistical Bureau: China Statistical Yearbook, China Statistical Publishing House, 1997.

investments on infrastructure building and staff training is an immediate concern. If some of them have less financing capacity, which seems inevitable, whether it will affect the quality of services and protection is another concern.

- *Covering the self-employed and workers of private firms.* A research report[11] prepared by the China Private Enterprises Study stated that as of 31 December 1997 the registered non-primary-industry self-employed entities accounted for 28 million, with 54 million workers, nearly two workers per unit, and there are 0.96 million private firms employing 13 million people, 14 workers per firm. In addition, there are thousands and millions of non-registered small businesses and workers. As elsewhere, to effectively cover this group scattered in an immense number of small work units always presents administrative difficulties and higher operating costs. According to the same report, 65 percent of private firms and 44 percent of self-employed entities are located in the eastern region of the country, the most economically developed area. Thus, it is more difficult for health insurance authorities in the regions to bring in this group. It may thus be wise not to include it in the initial phase. But as an increasing proportion of this group is made up of laid-off workers of the SOE, for social stability reasons this would not be politically acceptable.

- *The enforcement problem associated with a part of the SOE.* Of the 206 million urban workforce, 110 million were SOE workers and 27 million were SOE retirees[12] at the end of 1998. But it is estimated that about one-third to one-half of SOEs are loss-makers. For instance, as a whole, 59,000 SOEs of the secondary industry ran a deficit of Yuan 8,770 million as a result of poor performance in the first trimester of 1998 in comparison with a profit of Yuan 580 million in the same period of the preceding year.[13] However, for political and social reasons, many of them still have to be maintained in place. It is estimated that such controversial phenomena will continue to exist for at least a few years. Apparently, many loss-makers in the SOE sector cannot afford to pay contribution dues. If the scope of the non-payment is large, the duration is long and there is no other workable solution, it will be catastrophic for a health insurance scheme like the BHISFUWP, and it will not be able to continue to pay out benefits in full nor on time.

Actually, the new old-age and unemployment insurance schemes have been experiencing such difficulties since their establishment. The situation deteriorated in 1998. It is reported that, due to the Asian financial crisis and the deepening of SOE reform, the participation and contribution-making rates of these two systems are very low. Despite a number of administrative efforts made to reinforce compliance, only 73 percent and 56 percent of urban employees respectively have registered with the two systems. The contribution-paid rates for the former scheme is 90.6 percent as the average and 72 percent as the lowest. This led to current-year deficits occurring in 25 provinces, municipalities and autonomous regions, out of 31 in total.[14] To maintain benefit payments, the government urgently called for setting up emergency funds at each administrative level. The needed resources were derived from three sources: central and local government budgets, enterprises in general, and affected firms in particular, one-third each in principle. After one year, this strategy is working well in terms of securing benefit delivery, but it is difficult to continue because of enterprises' low capacity for making this sort of contribution, which obliged either the central or the local governments to make it up. In 1998, the central government alone allocated Yuan 16.8 billion to the emergency funds.[15] For 1999, the amount of allocation to the social security subsidy fund on the central government budget jumped 248.6 percent.[16] It is becoming a heavy financial burden to the government, because statistics show that the share of government revenues in GDP is declining to less than 11 percent of GDP in 1999, but that is normally as high as 20 percent and 30-40 percent respectively in developing and industrialized countries respectively. Given that, whether the central and local governments as a whole can continue to support this strategy, weighted by an additional subsidy to the BHISFUWP, is questionable. Without sufficient resources for paying benefits, personal coverage is meaningless.

- *Further extension to the rest of the urban population, approximately one-half the total urban population.* This group includes military personnel, university students, dependents of the insured and rural immigrants. The first two groups are currently covered by existing special arrangements; a part of the third category, mainly children, is entirely or partially insured under employer liability programs. Therefore, the first question here is whether to integrate the first three groups into the BHISFUWP or to replace the existing mechanisms by other institutional arrangements. However, as neither students nor children are income earners, it is difficult to open an IMA for them. As to the last group, in general they have no access so far to any formal health insurance protection. But it is a large category too; about 40 million people have now settled in cities for a relatively long time.[17] For this group, due to their high mobility tendency and unstable, sometimes unregistered, employment status, effective coverage is more difficult to achieve. However, for political and social reasons, they cannot be excluded for long either. That would also be a serious challenge to the government.

Funding: Is It Sufficient?

As mentioned above, the overall financing resources available for the BHISFUWP are equal to 8 percent of payroll plus government subsidies for administering the system. Therefore, this contribution rate is crucial for benefit delivery. According to a responsible official, this rate is determined on the basis of actual average health spending per worker per annum in the urban area in recent years, which accounts for about 8 percent of average salary.[18] By adding up government subsidies for administration, policymakers are convinced such a levy can comfortably assure that the system meets the demands for basic health care required by most insured persons.

In principle, the question of whether a contribution rate is appropriate can only be assessed in relation to the defined benefit package. That is why the contribution fixed at 2.64 percent of the payroll can still produce a large surplus in Thailand but is vastly insufficient in nearly all industrialized countries. It also depends on the demographic trend in the specific country, the age structure of the insured, the extent of personal coverage, the contribution base, etc. Previous expenditure figures alone cannot build up a solid and actuarial basis for determining and adjusting the contribution rate. Thus, some additional aspects need to be taken into account.

- *The negative aspect:*

Ageing population. This trend is much more rapid in China than in industrialized countries according to a recent study of the MOH.[19] It took 85 years and 115 years respectively for France and Sweden to double the number of elderly persons, but this happened in China in only 27 years. By the end of 1998, 120 million persons, equal to 10 percent of the total population, were aged 60 years and above. The number of elderly persons is estimated to reach 400 million in the middle of the next century. The life expectancy at birth[20] rose from 35 years in 1949 to 70.83 years in 1998. This demographic evolution would result in a rise in demand for health care and a rise in costs as well, whilst the proportion of economically active workers as contributors is diminishing.

Lower contribution base stipulated for laid-off workers and for the unemployed. As contributions paid on behalf of laid-off workers are calculated on the basis of 8 percent of 60 percent of regional average income, collectable revenues in this regard will be accordingly reduced. Mr. Li Boyong, the Minister of the MOL, claimed[21] on 9 March 1998 that by the end of 1997, except for the unemployed being 3 percent of the urban labor force, there were 11.5 million laid-off workers, equal to about 10 percent of the workforce in SOEs. It is anticipated about another 10 million redundant workers will be added in the period from 1999 to 2001. The large scope of this group implies that a considerable reduction in generated revenues both to the IMAs and to the HIPF would have adverse impacts on the laid-off workers themselves as well as the whole insured population. In particular, some regions such as Shanghai, Fuzhou, Zhengzhou, and Chengdou (where layoffs are massive—amounting to 14 percent, 27.5 percent, 14.8 percent, and 30 percent respectively of the total local workforce[22] in 1997) will definitely have more difficulty in running the scheme.

Anticipated low compliance rate. As mentioned in the preceding section, it is likely that contribution-paid rates of many SOEs will be insufficient in the case of the BHISFUWP as the macro environment remains roughly the same as last year.

Two-component structure and regulations on the use of resources. As the total revenues coming from employers' and workers' contributions are split into two parts, one to the IMAs, the other to the HIPF, and are also completely blocked in each component and even in each individual IMA, no funds can be transferred to trade off shortfalls elsewhere. As a consequence, this results in a reduction in the generated resources, represented by a formula: (3.8 percent + 4.2 percent) < 8 percent.

Regionally run arrangements. As each region is responsible for designing and operating its own BHISFUWP scheme, funds are also blocked within the territory of each region. Given the large disparities in the economy and in the age structure of the insured population between regions, the same contribution rate will make local schemes operated in a locality like Sheng Zheng in Guang Dong Province, which has both the highest income per capita and the lowest average age of residents in the country, much better off than those in the northeastern part of the country, for instance.

- *The favorable aspect:*

Special arrangements for privileged groups. Both decisions on maintaining the existing mechanisms for senior government officers, ex-cadres and war veterans, who are the most costly categories in terms of expenditure per capita, and on setting up supplementary schemes for civil servants would ease some financial pressure which would otherwise be imposed on the BHISFUWP.

Extending personal coverage to the non-SOE sector. Comparatively, the financing capacity of enterprises and employees in the non-SOE sector is higher, with a lower average workforce age. Thus, it is possible to obtain a higher contribution-paid rate from this sector. The weighted share of this sector, accounting for one-third of the urban workforce discussed above, makes this more meaningful. It is strongly believed that the momentum of growth in this sector is high and will be further reinforced because the National Assembly approved in March 1999[23] a favorable amendment to the National Constitution, which declares for the first time since 1949 that the private sector constitutes an important, rather than complementary, component of the economy. Thus, the effective inclusion of non-SOE workers will subsequently help to offset shortfalls occurring in the SOE sector for the reasons explained above.

Once the contribution rate has been determined on a sound actuarial basis, there is also a need to set up a reviewing mechanism to evaluate and adjust it regularly.

Benefit Package: Is It Adequate and Secured?

To the insured, an adequate and secured benefit package is the core concern. Since the defined benefits under the BHISFUWP are provided separately under the two tiers, it may be convenient to review them separately.

- Under the IMAs

There are two relevant figures concerning this matter: the maximum benefit up to 10 percent of average regional annual income, to which each insured person is in principle entitled, and the annual global allocation equal to about 3.8 percent of the payroll to the IMAs for financing defined benefit payments.

From the above figures, it can be seen at the macro level that a gap equal to 4.2 percent of the payroll exists between the designated benefit scope and the current year resources. However, this aggregate gap will be smaller in reality, because there will always be a part of the insured population in a given time who spend less than the average, and accumulated savings in personal IMAs can be carried over.

At the micro level, the situation is much more complicated due to a series of variants: (a) individual salary—according to the formulae, lower salaries lead to lower allocations to personal IMAs or vice versa; (b) the method adopted by a local scheme to distribute the part of employers' contributions, about 30 percent, to individual IMAs; (c) the health status of an insured person both in the current year and in preceding years; (d) the current year's expenditure on health care; (e) accumulated savings carried over from previous periods, etc. Apparently, these factors vary widely by person and by time, so when putting them against a uniform line (10 percent of average regional income as the maximum benefit payable under the IMA) the implications for each insured person would be considerably different.

For instance, assuming that part of the employers' contribution is redistributed at an even rate of 1.8 percent of an individual salary to each IMA, that there are no savings available in any personal IMA, and that everyone has consumed an amount up to the maximum line on health care in the given year, then the results would indicate that an insured person who earns 2.6 times or more the average regional income and whose health costs in this category are fully covered by the current year's allocation to his/her IMA (even if he/she always spends up to the maximum) would be very comfortable. Otherwise, some surplus will be accumulated in his/her account and never be used, except for cases in which his/her income is dramatically reduced or he/she dies. On the contrary, the annual income in an individual IMA can only cover 38 percent or 19 percent respectively of the full cost, and if the insured's wages are equal to the average or less, half of it. Unfortunately, the health status of the cohort of low-income workers is generally inferior in reality to that of their superior colleagues. Once an insured person falls into the category of low income with poor health, he/she may either choose to delay or cancel necessary treatment thus causing a deterioration in his/her health, but if the insured person does seek treatment, the result may be subsequent financial hardship.

Thus, there is an important need for putting into place some global measures to mitigate or minimize the adverse impacts. In fact, even within the current structure, it is possible to do so. One possibility is to lower the 10 percent line or to align it with individual income rather than with the average regional revenue. Since the actual average health spending per capita in urban areas in recent years is only around 8 percent of average income, this 10 percent line appears too high. Another possibility is to make the redistribution of the defined employers' contribution in favor of vulnerable groups. Some of these approaches have already been used in Hai Nan Province during the piloting period. A further option is that the rest of the health bills are picked up by the HIPF once the amount of pocket payment under the IMA tier exceeds a certain percent of the insured person's annual income. This method has also been widely adopted in previous years' reforming exercises.

- *Under the HIPF*

Except for the imposition of a threshold and a ceiling, medical benefits provided under this component are not much different from a normal health insurance scheme. Potential concerns associated with the first line have just been analyzed. It is advisable to enlarge the responsibility scope of the HIPF as much as possible by lowering this line. This will immediately improve the quality of protection for vulnerable groups when other factors remain the same.

Comparatively, concerns are more linked with the top line, because the potential financial pressure under the IMA is limited within the said 10 percent line, which is relatively bearable for the insured persons. But this is certainly not the case for certain serious treatments, such as cancer cures and organ transplants. It is not unusual for these treatments to cost more than six to ten times the average regional income, which is not feasible for many families.

Therefore, the hope is then placed on the establishment of supplementary schemes. Taxation advantage is accorded accordingly. Some pilot schemes have been reported too. For example, the city of Xia Men in Fu Jian Province[24] jointly launched a complementary health insurance program by the local government and a commercial insurance company. A total of 240,000 persons were registered in 1998, of which 317 received benefits amounting to Yuan 4 million, and the highest single payment was about Yuan 105,000. Nevertheless, it is doubtful that China can set up a complementary mechanism with wide enough coverage in the medium term. For one reason, the new system is just starting, and much remains to be done. Therefore, supplementary schemes are not a top priority. Secondly, the commercial health insurance market is much less developed in China. Thirdly, facing the market competition, many employers are less willing to make or not capable of making extra contributions.

Given the above, it is advisable for the government to first establish the expenditure structure by person and by year to estimate how many insured will exceed that limit, how heavy it is in relation to the individual regular income, and whether it is possible to lower the threshold and increase the ceiling. No doubt, this should be considered on an actuarial evaluation basis.

Cost Containment: Is It Efficient?

Among the fundamental problems facing the old health insurance system since economic reform, especially since the late 1980s, is the spiralling of rising costs in terms of total health spending in GDP and in terms of health spending per capita in real terms. Statistics show that the former increased from 2.9 percent in 1978 and 3.0 percent in 1986 to 3.8 percent in 1993, whilst the latter rose to an average 8 percent per annum for the 1978-86 period and then accelerated to 11 percent for 1986-93, but the real GDP per capita grew only 7.7 percent per annum over the two periods. Expenditure figures by groups suggest two urban health insurance schemes actually contributed much more to this increase. For instance, between 1981 and 1993, per capita health spending in rural areas increased from Yuan 21 to Yuan 60, while under the government insurance system it increased from Yuan 96 to Yuan 389.[25]

Such excessive cost escalation is commonly considered unaffordable and constitutes one of the basic causes for the eventual failure of the old health insurance regime. To avoid committing the same error and to secure benefit payments to the insured, the government has placed great emphasis on cost containment, and a series of measures ranging from the two-tier structure to health sector reform have been taken for this purpose.

But many international studies show that with a different approach some countries have done better than others in controlling health care costs without harming access and health outcomes. For instance, in 1960 Japan and the USA all spent 3-5.5 percent of their national income on health, a share similar to what China spends today. But spending rates diverged sharply over the next 30 years, with health spending reaching 14 percent of GDP in the USA by 1993—even though 15 percent of its population is still uninsured. By contrast, Japan spent only 7.3 percent of GDP on health in 1993, with nearly universal coverage and the world's highest life expectancy.[26]

Therefore, two points should be kept in mind. First, there is a worldwide pattern of overall expenditure on health care rising faster than GDP, especially following demographic changes and continuing economic growth, because the population needs and is able and willing to invest more in its health. Here, some external factors are beyond the control of the scheme. The World Bank estimates[27] the factor of the ageing population alone will increase health spending in China from 3.2 percent of GDP in 1992 to 5 percent in 2010 and 7 percent by 2030. Secondly, cost containment is just a means but not an ultimate objective of the system, so it should not be achieved at the expense of access to health services and of the health of the insured population.

When looking into concrete measures on cost control taken inside and outside the health insurance system, such as the introduction of the IMA, co-payment by the insured, the threshold and ceiling lines for HIPF benefits, limiting the number of hospitals an insured is allowed to choose as his/her health provider, separating medical services and drug selling, etc., there is impressive weight putting on the demand side. In the preceding sections, potential problems in this regard have already been explored. Despite certain undesirable implications some measures have on vulnerable groups, the possibility of escaping cost controls still exists. For example, apart from emergencies and serious illness, an insured can concentrate medical treatments in a year when the balance accumulated in his/her IMA is high enough to cover the designated cost. This is similar to the situation in Switzerland, where an insured can choose a suitable benefit threshold with a particular premium rate for each year in line with his/her projection and personal planning. In addition, if no complementary program is in place, it is still possible to spread the overall estimated costs over two years or more under the current fee-for-service payment system.

On the supply side, cost control measures are apparently weak. In particular, a provider payment mechanism more efficient than a fee-for-service system such as the capitation payment system is still absent. Experience gained worldwide suggests a good provider payment system is more crucial and more important for cost containment, because it is the doctor who is the active conductor during the course of treatment, while the patient is more passive. A doctor's opinion has a strong influence on the patient. Furthermore, it is also the doctor who professionally knows the possible treatments and their cost. For their own interests, health care providers tend to propose an expensive treatment or to over-provide health services. A fee-for-service payment system makes this very easy to realize. But this is not the case for a capitation payment mechanism. As the fee-for-service payment system is still in use in the case of the BHISFUWP, providers will thus have flexibility within the limited scope of the HIPF to over-prescribe medical services. It is true that the introduction of an IMA and its very nature make a capitation payment system difficult to be adopted. However, some aggregate prepayment approaches, like the one used in Zhenjiang City of Jiangsu Province during the piloting period, are worth consideration.

Finally, it should be pointed out that some savings accumulated in many individual IMAs will never be used, which represents a resource waste. Unfortunately, this fact has not yet attracted due attention of the Chinese policymakers.

Health Sector Reform: Is It Harmonized?

The public health sector serves as the main health service provider for the insured; its reform is therefore important and indispensable for the success of the BHISFUWP.

Almost all problems of this sector having direct or indirect impacts on the new health insurance system derive from a dramatic change in its financing method, i.e., from "full subsidy financing" to "partial subsidy financing." In the past, like all other public institutions, hospitals and other medical institutions were fully financed by the government or the SOEs. This is why under the old regime there was no direct interest or motivation for hospital managers to seek revenues from patients, and they were not concerned about the price level of various medical items determined by the Price Committee of the State Council. During that time, particularly in the 1960s and 1970s, the price was frequently used by the government as a policy tool to increase access to health care: prices on medical visits and hospital stays were reduced so that a poor peasant could afford them. As a result, prices for most medical services, especially with considerable labor input, have dropped considerably below actual producing costs and have also been frozen for a long time.

Since economic reform, like other government institutions, public hospitals and other medical institutions have to generate a growing part of their total revenue to cover operating costs, which is now up to 85 percent, whilst government subsidies are accordingly diminishing. Table 5.3 provides more details. In parallel with the change of the financing approach, the government introduced two methods for hospital managers to generate needed income: a makeup of 15 percent of the price at both the wholesale and the retail level and fewer or no price controls on high technology tests. Meanwhile, the prices on basic health services were maintained to ensure the population a minimum access to health care. In order to generate a small profit to cross-subsidize under-priced health services, hospitals had to oversell a high volume of drugs, which were not only purchased outside from manufacturers but also produced inside. They equally over-purchased, over-installed and over-provided high-technology diagnostic tests for the same reasons. Subsequently, this has substantially distorted the pattern of medical services with over-provision and under-provision of others. For instance, drug purchases account for 52 percent of health spending in China, compared with an average of 14 percent in OECD countries and 15-40 percent in most other developing countries.[28] Associated with the distortion of the medical price structure and the need for income, the behavior and morality of medical professionals have been somehow distorted, and the quality of the medical service as a whole has been adversely affected, too.

To address these problems and to facilitate the establishment of the BHISFUWP, the government has started to accelerate the reform in the health sector through all the measures illustrated above, including disciplining medical personnel, separating pharmaceutical sales from hospital services, readjusting price structures, and introducing competitive mechanisms. Certainly, these reform measures will help but will not be sufficient. As long as health providers have to cover most of the operational costs and no provider payment system with a strong cost-containment effect is introduced to replace the current fee-for-service payment mechanism (whether or not the health service price structure is readjusted and drug selling is separate) over-providing health services to the insured patients, including those with high professional inputs once their prices have been increased, will always be a serious problem to a health insurance scheme. Therefore, having an aggregate prepayment mechanism in place is vital to the BHISFUWP.

Table 5. 3
Government Subsidies Earmarked to Public Hospitals
1995

	Actual amount (Yuan 100 million)
1. Government subsidy	75.5
on retirement pension	33.6
on staff payroll	41.9
2. The overall payroll	173.3
subsidy as % of the overall payroll	24.2%

Source: Ministry of Public Health: *Public health sector reform and development*, Series Study No.1, Beijing, 1996.

Concern also arises from the decision on increasing the prices of those under-cost products and services with high labor input as envisaged in the decree. As these prices have been largely below the real cost for a long time, the extent of the increase must be accordingly substantial. On the other hand, no proportional cuts on drug and high-tech test prices are foreseen, which may be due to some political considerations on the development of pharmaceutical and medical instrument-producing industries and services. Consequently, this price adjustment may push up the overall price on health care and result in costs rising on the balance sheet of the BHISFUWP.

Clearly, the health sector stands not just as a health provider for the insured population but also for the uninsured population. It is a challenge for the government to accommodate the insured, the uninsured and the health provider at the same time. It is not entirely clear at the moment about the future policy on securing the uninsured population a minimum access to health care services, and the reform in the health sector is far from that goal, but it is certain that any changes will have some impact, direct or indirect, on the BHISFUWP.

Governance: Is It Reinforced?

It appears that the governance model applied to the BHISFUWP is somewhat similar to that implemented in the United Kingdom and Ireland. In other words, responsibility lies, in general, with the government, and there is little opportunity for the social partners to influence policy or control the management of the system. However, as it is run in each region, responsibility and power for policymaking are therefore shared between the central government and local governments. It is the central government which determines national policy and guidelines, while it is the local governments which apply these national rules to their schemes with necessary modifications in line with their situation. In the future, this may result in a considerable policy disparity between regions that will be reflected on personal coverage, benefit provision, contribution rates, etc. Thus, promoting the pooling level and eventually unifying the system in the future will be difficult. At the policy level, no consultation mechanism on a regular basis is envisaged in the decree, although trade unions and employers' organizations will be invited to make comments from time to time on the government's policy proposals. This is actually consistent with the relatively low level of the development of both workers' and employers' organizations in the country.

At the institutional level, operational institutions are not accorded autonomous status and corresponding powers, because they are still closely attached to the government and regarded as semi-government organs. But there is an increasing call for detaching them and making them into non-profit-making establishments with some autonomous power. As to the BHISFUWP, the extent of its functioning and influence would differ from region to region.

At the operational level, there is much to be done in the initial phase. Reinforcing governance at this level, including staff training, is the immediate task for the local authorities.

Conclusion

From the above, we now know what the BHISFUWP looks like, its features, strengths, weaknesses and potential problems. But at this early stage of the establishment of the new schemes, this chapter does not intend to offer a panoramic picture of the new system; nor is it an assessment of the system's feasibility, efficiency and effectiveness. What this chapter explores and analyses is rather preliminary and theoretical, given the fact that the new system has not yet been implemented and that considerable modifications are expected to be made in both the designing and operating phases by the local authorities.

For outside observers, the most impressive two characteristics of the new system are its two-tier structure and extensive personal coverage. No doubt, thanks to this legal provision on coverage, all workers in the formal sector and some in the informal sector as well will be insured, whether adequately or not, under the BHISFUWP. Two large groups are the main beneficiaries: one is the non-SOE workers who were previously excluded and the other is a part of SOE workers who could not, partially or even entirely, receive promised benefits due to financial difficulties their employers experienced. A similar move in coverage is rarely seen in other developing countries.

As regards the two-tier structure, some potential problems and shortcomings associated with it have been noted in the preceding sections. But it is not a pure provident fund, nor is it a pure health insurance. It is somewhat a hybrid of the two: half social insurance, half provident fund; half solidarity, half self-reliance. By combining the two halves into a whole to make full use of the strengths of each, the Chinese are trying to better adapt the new system to the changing world and to provide the population with sustainable health protection. In fact, if the BHISFUWP is seen in a broader perspective, it will be seen that it does not stand alone; its structure and nature are inherently consistent with both the new old-age insurance system and the socialist market economy. This constitutes a new identity for the Chinese community in the changing world. It seems changes cannot be made only to a part of the new identity, the two-tier structure of the BHISFUWP, for example, without corresponding changes to the other parts.

In conclusion, whether the new health insurance system succeeds or fails, its potential implications for the population and the economy will be significant. Given the population size of the country and the possibility that its influence on the development of health insurance may go beyond national borders, in particular in those economies in transition or in the region, it is advisable for the international health insurance community to observe more closely its development and constructively assist the Chinese authorities in improving the system if needed.

Notes

1. In conformity with the Resolution on Social Security Reform approved by the 15th National Assembly of the Communist Party, on 14 December 1998, the State Council in Beijing issued a decree (No. 44/1998) setting up a Basic Health Insurance System for Urban Working People (BHISFUWP), laying down the basic legal and policy framework for establishing a new health protection mechanism for urban employees. It is envisaged that from the year 2000 the BHISFUWP will start to be implemented nationwide on a regional basis following a one-year designing exercise.
2. *People's Daily*, 14 April 1999, Beijing.
3. Ibid., 1 March 1999, Beijing, China. But in line with the *China Statistical Yearbook 1997* (Beijing, China Statistical Publishing House), the population accounted for 1,223 million by the end of 1996; 198 million are urban workers. Of these, 112 million are SOE workers, 30 million COE workers, 23 million self-employed and private enterprises employees, and 9 million workers employed in the other ownership units. Also, in 1996, China had 32 million retirees, of which 24 million are ex-workers of state and collective enterprises and 10 million urban unemployed. Even taking into account some changes which have occurred in the labor market in China since 1997, it is still difficult to understand how this coverage of 13 percent was calculated, which is inconsistent with the relative provisions stipulated in the decree and the actual figures.
   The majority of this group are redundant workers of SEOs who used to hold a working-life employment contract. To facilitate them to adapt themselves to the new situation in the labor market, they are allowed to enter a re-employment center

instead of registering immediately with an unemployment insurance scheme. They lose their job but receive reduced incomes from the re-employment center for up to three years, during which they keep all entitlements to enterprise-based welfare benefits as usual and are remained on the lists of workers of their previous employers. If they cannot find a job within that three-year period, they will subsequently be transferred to an unemployment insurance fund and treated as a normal unemployed person after that.

5. Ibid., 1 March 1999, Beijing.
6. Statement of State Statistical Bureau, Beijing, reported in *People's Daily*, 6 October 1998, Beijing.
7. *Financing health care: Issues and options for China*, World Bank, 1997, Washington, DC.
8. *China Statistical Yearbook 1997*, Beijing, China Statistical Informational and Consultancy Service Centre.
9. *Government Bulletin on the Statistics of Economic and Social Development in 1998*, PRC, 26 February 1999, Beijing.
10. *People's Daily*, 8 February 1999, Beijing.
11. Ibid., 8 March 1999, Beijing.
12. *Government Bulletin on the Statistics of Economic and Social Development in 1998*, op. cit.
13. *United Morning News*, 16 June 1998, Singapore.
14. National Conference on Expanding Social Insurance Coverage and Strengthening Compliance, held by the Government of PRC on 26 February 1999 in Beijing.
15. *Report on the Performance of the Government Budget in 1998* and *Proposal for the 1999 Budget*, the Ministry of Finance, PRC, Beijing.
16. *The Performance of the State Budget in the First Trimester of 1999*, the Ministry of Finance, PRC, Beijing.
17. Hua Xia Wen Zhai Regular, April 1999. Internet Address: www.cnd.org:8006/HXWZ.
18. *People's Daily*, 1 March 1999, Beijing.
19. Ibid., 8 April 1999, Beijing.
20. Ibid., 5 April 1999, Beijing.
21. Ibid., 9 March 1998, Beijing.
22. Hua Xia Wen Zhai Regular. February 1998. Internet Address: www.cnd.org:8006/HXWZ
23. Amendment to the National Constitution, approved by the Parliament, reported by *People's Daily*, 17 March 1999, Beijing.
24. *People's Daily*, 1 March 1999, Beijing.
25. *Financing health care: Issues and options for China*, op. cit.
26. Ibid.
27. Ibid.
28. Ibid.

Part 4

Refining Benefits to Meet Current Needs

6

Moving to Integrate Prevention, Curative Prevention, and Curation

K. Spyra, T. Hansmeier, and W. Müller-Fahrnow

Prevention, rehabilitation and cure are three concepts of health care, whose significance for the whole system must be obvious even to the layman. If one analyzes the substance, one very quickly stumbles on a dilemma caused by the ambiguity of the definition and practical management of health care, which from a practical point of view can best be formally clarified by reference back to Germany's social legislation and its interpretation in the provision of health insurance benefits. As soon as one seeks the reasons for the many alleged deficiencies in the reality of care provision, it at once becomes clear that this approach is not adequate, and here we come up against not only weaknesses in practical delivery but also gaps in the state of scientific knowledge.

The methodological problem in defining the content of the three concepts in a meaningful way—apart from ubiquitous differences of opinion in the scientific disciplines concerning the formation of each concept as a problem of canonization of relative truths—lies in the actual reality of the organization of health care. The process of health (and social) care is by its nature a continuous and complex integral whole. Every division into time, content or other unit may be useful on scientific (theoretical explanation) or practical (organization of delivery) grounds, but it is also open to analysis based on the viewpoint of particular interests.

The "artificial" breakdown of the continuity of care is always a problem when the original objectives are not achieved, especially if there are practical deficiencies in care, whose scientific explanation is impeded by entrenched concepts and, worse still, established institutionalized authorities. There have been signs of this situation for years in the German health care system, which despite its many successes also shows serious defects. The problem of integration of prevention, rehabilitation and cure, addressed here, could be described in the broadest sense by the catch phrase "demarcation problems." In Germany, historically, a divided social security system has grown up, in which responsibility for different parts of what was originally an integrated social service by law (Social Code) was divided between various institutions. The interplay of the historically evolved reality and the provisions of social legislation led to a degree of distortion in practice, which can be analyzed on three levels:

1.   the first concerns the theoretical scientific questions of a structure of the whole care process which makes sense in analytical and/or organizational terms.

2.   based on this, the adequacy of the legal and administrative structure must be analyzed.

3.   lastly, using the knowledge of the implications for care acquired from the analyses in (1) and (2), management strategies, among others, in the broadest sense, must be modified.

The framework of the following report is based on this three-pronged approach. The theoretical problems of the concepts of prevention, rehabilitation and cure should be first outlined on the basis of the global approach of the World Health Organization (WHO) definitions, in relation to the German health system. Even the presentation of the practical defects in health care systems is confined in a relatively global sense to the macro-view of the rehabilitation system and again to a few core issues.

The focal point of the chapter is the presentation of a methodological approach—the so-called Rehabilitanden-Management-Kategorien (RMK) (Rehabilitation-Management-Category) approach to the practical integration of prevention, rehabilitation and cure. The example of cardiology shows how changes in acute medicine affect the needs and regulation of access to rehabilitation and what this means in terms of the need for quality management in rehabilitative care.

Prevention, Rehabilitation, and Cure—The Problem of Integration from the Theoretical Standpoint

If one looks in the literature for a meaning of the concepts of prevention, rehabilitation and cure, one finds as many definitions as authors.

The lack of conceptual clarity, however, merely reflects the fundamental problems in reality: health care must be understood as geared to the "whole man" in his bio-psycho-social dimensions only as an integral, complex and continuous process. Against this background, different definitions of these terms seek to pick out individual aspects of the content, method or time frame, on which it seems useful to focus for practical or theoretical reasons. The efforts at the stage of defining concepts, especially the breakdown of their content, are already symptomatic of the underlying indivisibility of the task.

We cannot go into all the nuances of the conceptual debate here. As a global approach only the WHO concept should be pursued. For this reason, the problem of the inherent ambiguities in the classification of practical operational areas in the German care system should be explained and a fundamental conceptual understanding be established for the following exposition.

The basis of the WHO concept is the schematic distinction of a (temporal) sequence of states of health, congenital disease, illness and impairment, disability and handicap. Under this model, a distinction is drawn between the concepts of primary, secondary and tertiary prevention on the basis of the stage of illness and the target group:[1] *primordial prevention* is thus the stage of prevention, which in relation to research into cardiac and circulatory disease was the last to be distinguished and is still little known today. It is based on social, economic and cultural conditions, which are known to contribute to higher risk of disease. The approach thus embraces all areas of life of the whole population and comes into play even before any symptoms of illness. Primary prevention concerns above all social policy programs in the broadest sense, in relation to coronary disease, for example, healthy nutrition, anti-smoking, regular physical exercise and prevention of high blood pressure.

The aim of *primary prevention* is to reduce the incidence of illness, by attacking the cause of illness and the corresponding risk factors. Primary prevention is thus effective even before an illness appears. It consists essentially of two strategies, which reflect two etiological standpoints. It can focus on the whole population and try to limit the global risk, or it can target individuals, whose constitution places them at exceptionally high risk.

In the German health insurance system, the approach to prevention is often confined to the WHO concept of primary prevention. This is connected to the way social legislation allocates responsibility for these areas, in that the law primarily and explicitly leaves it in the hands of health insurance.

A further stage of prevention under the WHO concept comes into play when the state of illness has arisen. The aim of *secondary prevention* is, by early recognition and timely treatment to cure the patient and limit any serious after effects of the illness. Secondary prevention thus comes in the time interval between the start of the illness and diagnosis. In other words, secondary prevention reduces the prevalence of illness in a population, by reducing its duration and consequences. In medical terms, it thus mainly falls within the traditional activities of treatment and therapy. However, it is not only (secondary) preventative and curative activities, at least in part, that necessarily belong together in the medical treatment process. Rehabilitation also has elements of secondary prevention: measures to minimize risk factors are, for example, a key component of rehabilitation, as is currently practiced in Germany.

Secondary prevention activities are thus an essential component of both cure and rehabilitation—the only difference being the primary objective: while the cure, in the narrowest sense, seeks to eliminate the causes of the illness and rehabilitation targets the after effects of illness, prevention is predicated on early treatment and thus on limitation of the related after effects of the illness. It is already clear from this that the conceptual ambiguities between cure, rehabilitation and (secondary) prevention stem from the indivisibility of the corresponding activities in the treatment process. Early diagnosis not only improves the chances of a cure, but also thereby allows the after effects of the illness to be kept to a minimum.

The WHO concept of *tertiary prevention* also hinges on prevention of illness. With its help, the progress of an illness can be stemmed or the appearance of complications in existing illnesses can be restricted. It particularly targets the consequences of illness, such as by measures to limit damage and disabilities, to alleviate pain caused by health problems and to help patients with incurable diseases to adjust. Tertiary prevention is thus both an important element of therapy/treatment on the one hand and of rehabilitation, on the other. The relevance of rehabilitation according to the WHO concept particularly concerns the management of the effects of illness, especially in the case of chronic illness. Even in the case of tertiary prevention, it is clearly difficult in practice to distinguish between preventive activities and treatment or rehabilitation, as one of the most important aims of the treatment of chronic illness in acute medicine is to prevent recurrence, and of rehabilitation to avoid (prevention) further damage to health or subsequent illness, which could arise from progress of the illness or from disabilities.

In the German health insurance scheme, the medical treatment element of *cure in the narrowest sense* is often called *acute medicine*. The legislation describes the activities of acute medicine as the stage between prevention and rehabilitation and makes the medical insurance sector responsible for this area. This gives the impression that the three areas of prevention, acute medicine and rehabilitation can be separated, with sequential activities, to be carried out by different agencies and thus with different organizational arrangements (institutions, concepts, etc.). Reliance on the conceptual significance of prevention and cure according to the WHO concept supports the emphasis here on the interrelated aspects.

If one takes the legal definition of the concept of rehabilitation in the German health insurance scheme, it encompasses both the WHO secondary and tertiary prevention stages. Although the content of rehabilitation like all concepts in social legislation is loosely defined, thus leaving room for specific definitions in individual cases, it can nevertheless be concluded that it is broadly directed at the consequences of illness and includes both secondary and tertiary preventative measures. While the legislator has handed responsibility for rehabilitation of bodily and motor damage (impairment), regardless of its social or professional consequences, exclusively to medical insurance, pensions insurance must intervene in rehabilitation in the event of a (threatened or actual) reduction in capacity to work. The bald alleviation of hardship caused by illness and the avoidance of dependency are not the legal responsibility of pensions insurance, although in practice they must for the most part be exercised in parallel. One of the reasons for this is that it is virtually impossible to carry out rehabilitation measures for disabled people in isolation from medical treatment.

With regard to the definition of the thematic concepts "prevention, rehabilitation and cure," this means that a strict distinction or delimitation of "curative" and "rehabilitative" therapies on the one hand, and preventative measures on the other, cannot be strictly sustained either in terms of content, or method or time. It is simply a difference of objectives and emphasis. In another sense, therefore, cure can also be understood as the umbrella concept, embracing the medical tasks of prevention, acute medicine and rehabilitation. Although this conceptualization seems to make sense in terms of the overall nature of the process, it is not to be further developed here. Bearing in mind the existing division and the related use of language in the German health insurance scheme, care should be understood in the narrower sense of acute medicine, and differentiated from prevention as the medical task of precautionary health care and rehabilitation as managing the consequences of illness. What problems of provision this legal differentiation of tasks might give rise to in practice will be briefly described below. The analysis is based on the authors' experiences from a technical rehabilitation angle.

"Demarcation Problems" in the German Health Insurance Scheme—An Analysis from a Technical Rehabilitation Angle

A particular feature of the German social security system is the division of responsibilities between different agencies. This relates both to the above-mentioned three areas of prevention, cure and rehabilitation, and to the various types of delivery within the rehabilitation system itself. This differentiation of agency fundamentally breaches the principle of integrated risk management: the service is delivered by the responsible social security agency, which also bears the risk of breakdown. Taking the example of pensions insurance, this means that it provides rehabilitation benefits when—and only when—the insured's capacity to work is endangered by illness or disability and there is a threat of early retirement from work (and thus payment of a pension). Acute medical and preventive measures in the narrower sense are explicitly excluded by the law from the responsibility of pensions insurance (except for rehabilitation measures for exceptionally dangerous employments) and included under health insurance. In addition to pensions insurance and health insurance, there are yet other providers of rehabilitation services, which cannot be covered in detail here. This division of tasks for health care in general and rehabilitation in particular between different agencies is, partly, something that has grown up historically and has led to each agency building up its own specialist field of competency. Thus pensions insurers, for example, mainly provide inpatient rehabilitation and have achieved a very high level of quality, which is internationally recognized, while in contrast the health insurance institutions concentrate on outpatient care. In the case of acute medicine, on the other hand, they provide both outpatient and inpatient care and in recent years have maintained a constant improvement.

At the same time, there have been increasingly frequent complaints both by those affected and by experts of a number of serious failings in the German health insurance scheme in general in recent years. This is especially true in relation to rehabilitation, a result of the lack of integration of the various services, caused by among other things the variety of agencies (Rehabilitation Commission[2], Commission of Enquiry for Concerted Action in the Health System,[3] *inter alia*). Just recently, at the 102nd German Doctors' Congress (2-4 June 1999 in Berlin), it was unanimously agreed by the delegates that: "instead of a dovetailing of acute medicine and rehabilitation, there is a discrepancy between curative and rehabilitative medical treatment. Effective, and thus cost-effective, early rehabilitation is often, therefore, unachievable." A need for treatment, however, was perceived within the rehabilitation system: "instead of working together, rehabilitation institutions increasingly isolate themselves from each other. The areas of responsibility and the length of administrative procedures are incomprehensible to doctors and patients¼instead of binding global standards for all agencies, there are at any one time individual concepts of quality targets, funding and perceived needs."[4]

The problem of internal and external demarcation lines in the rehabilitation system, for many years a subject of criticism, have become more acute under the pressure of various recent social changes. These changes include the demographic ageing of the population, the change in the landscape of illness, marked in particular by the increase in chronic illnesses and an expansion of the concepts of illness through greater differentiation between pathological conditions, earlier diagnosis and expansion of diagnostic and therapeutic capabilities; the expansion of pharmaceutical and technical treatment strategies; a change in social values in the direction of growing priority to "good health"; the trend towards globalization of health risks as a result of the international ecological crisis; the increase in social inequality; the change in health care from extending life to improving the quality of life.

This and other processes are taking place against a background of society's increased resource constraints, which results on the one hand in the traditional problems of health care becoming more acute and on the other to a greater monetary or economic element in the discussion.[5] The focus of attention on the "money" issue is not only confined to social policy discussions, but is increasingly heard in the choice of strategies and instruments for driving the related processes. The latest example of this trend is the introduction in acute medicine of flat rates per case and in rehabilitation the global budget ceiling (since 1997) through the so-called growth and employment productivity law. Neither approach built into its financial arrangements any provision for a reduction of existing deficits and has to some extent even increased them. The introduction of flat rates for cases in acute medicine, including rejection at the demarcation lines between acute medicine and rehabilitation have been criticized because of the danger of a fall in quality of care, such as through unacceptable curtailment of acute treatment and early transfer to rehabilitation; a tendency towards risk selection in patients, which leads, among other things, to increased numbers of operations in the face of doubtful symptoms and an undesirable shifting of responsibility for treatment (shuffling patients). Moreover, case flat rates have not led to the dismantling of demarcation lines, but have rather sharpened them. Against the background of the legislation to shrink the rehabilitation budget, as in other statutory structural measures in this area (for example by shortening the normal period of rehabilitation from four to three weeks), there is a serious danger for the quality of care. With ever more patients in the acute medicine area now undergoing surgery, and being moved more quickly into rehabilitation where, having been inadequately prepared for the rehabilitative phase, they are supposed to be rehabilitated in a shorter time, the problems of quality of care are clearly at the forefront.

When financial strategies are thus clearly inadequate, at least in the foreseeable future, to solve the care deficit in health systems generally and in the border areas in particular, then the question arises as to what alternatives, with their related strategies, must be developed from a technical rehabilitation angle.

Quality Management as a Strategic Approach to the Integration of Prevention, Rehabilitation, and Cure

It is generally considered that the prime aim of all management approaches to the health system is quality. Such strategies must therefore take this aspect as priority, because there is no escaping the fact that quality will not be achieved by self-regulation. This statement applies particularly to the peculiarities of the health market.[6] Unlike in non-health industry and services, there is no question here of a free market, with free supply and demand, but a mixture of private and state regulated supply. The need for regulatory intervention is based on the absence of significant bases for a free market economy in the health sector. By this is meant, for example, such preconditions for the free market as all participants having complete information, the principle of scale, including the existence of a sufficiently large number of suppliers and the openness of the market to change, for example, through an absence of entry and exit barriers for all participants. In contrast to this (and other) free market conditions, there is an extremely skewed distribution of information, in this case knowledge, in the health market, which favors the typical doctor. The doctor has a significant knowledge advantage, since the patient clearly cannot define the health objective of treatment, nor foresee when and in what context the need for treatment will come into play.

These and other peculiarities mean that quality in the health sector does not automatically flow from a free play between supply and demand, but needs targeted regulations. In the current German health insurance scheme it is clear that the quality and costs of medical care are mainly determined by doctors' groups and pharmaceutical and medical equipment industries, and assured by the doctors' monopoly over the definition of how to measure quality. Despite democratic regulations, the consumers have little scope for influence. Under the current legal and political arrangements, the so-called intermediary organizations, such as pensions and medical insurance institutions, have been given a structural and moderating role to ensure that quality is measured in a rational way, based on real scientific grounds and not on the monopoly of the health provider.

The social problems described above give rise to demands on the health system, which cannot be managed by financial or structural measures alone, but need quality-oriented treatment strategies. The effect of the increasing awareness of these demands, originating in the USA, is a growing pursuit of modern quality management in Germany, too. Alongside attempts at theoretical problem solving, interest is focusing on a variety of core strategic organizational measures. The buzz phrases include concepts such as Total Quality Management (TQM), the so-called 5 point-program of the German Pensions Insurance for Quality Assurance in medical rehabilitation and the EFQM concept. From a methodological point of view, these programs start with similar strategic goals, where the focus lies on specific instrumental and procedural arrangements. The measures taken up to now primarily emphasize two key points:

1.   the interactive component, i.e., the development and use of modern organizational concepts.

2.   the outcome-oriented component, i.e., scientifically based evaluation of the quality of the structure, process and result.

At the center, at the borderline, as it were, of both approaches, lies the pursuit of *quality standards* in health care. As scientifically based guidelines for the quality of care, they are appropriate for regulation of treatment and thus to promote high quality treatment. Since the launch in the USA, back in the early 1990s, of a government initiative for a scientifically based development of guidelines in the form of so-called PORTs (Patient Outcome Research Teams),[7] there has been a consensus in the German health system that medical guidelines must be envisaged as a sensible and necessary decision-making aid in ensuring high quality medical care. Despite numerous developments in this area, there has nevertheless been repeated doubt cast on the quality of a large part of the guidelines published in the German language. "In recent years, several hundred guidelines from specialist associations and their *ad hoc* expert groups have been published in a frantic short-term approach, in content more like text books and the collected experience of handed down tradition than true standard-setting on a scientific basis." (E. Buchhorn, 50th Bavarian Medical Conference 1997, quoted from Leitlinien-In-Fo[8]). This is, however, an international problem. Against this background, the Federal Medical Council and National Health Doctors' Association established their joint position in 1997 in "Evaluation criteria for guidelines in medical care" (Federal Medical Council, 1997). These "guidelines on guidelines" reflect both national and international views of the nature of "good" guidelines (Institute of Medicine 1990, AWMF 1996, Canadian Medical Association 1993). Without going here into all the requirements of guidelines, available in a checklist from the above-mentioned institutions for the German health insurance scheme, a central point should be noted. The value of the recommendations in the guidelines depends on the degree to which they are scientifically based. The most valuable guidelines are those characterized, at the least, by a random, controlled study, while the least valuable are treatment standards supported only by expert opinions.

When one considers further that in the German rehabilitation system it is almost impossible to achieve the highest level of evidence from randomized clinical studies on ethical grounds (under existing medical and insurance legislation, a legally guaranteed service to the insured cannot be refused on the groups of research), the question arises of alternatives for the clearest way of setting target standards. In this connection, the experience in the development of flat rates for cases or case-groups in acute medicine should be noted.

Treatment Standards—Methodological Requirements for Effective Management Tools and Their Expression in a Scientific Rehabilitation System in Rehabilitation-Management Categories (RMK)

The above-mentioned deficiencies in care in relation to the introduction of flat rates for cases can be attributed to significant defects in the structuring of the underlying groups. With either a one-sided "bottom up" (Germany) or "top down" approach (USA) to the construction of groups,[9] i.e., either exclusively expert definitions without sufficient empirical evaluation or one-sided empirical inference on the basis of less selected or standardized cases without sufficient scientific evaluation, the necessary harmonization of performance and costs cannot be achieved.

These weaknesses stem from a central methodological dilemma in determining the treatment standards specific to each group: the "products" of health care, unlike industrial products, can only be homogenous in statistical terms. A precise standardization of performance parameters or their classification as typical for treatment standards is not possible in the context of the genuinely individual nature of the treatment of each case. The degree of homogeneity of case groups can in these conditions only be a compromise between the practicability of the classification on the one hand and individual precision on the other.

Performance specifications in terms of case-group specific treatment standards can also only cover typical cases and are not, therefore, necessarily relevant to individual cases. The methodological dilemma of a theory-based setting of treatment standards on the one hand and the practical reflection of specific individual treatment on the other can only be resolved epistemologically by an iterative process. Such a process is needed, in order gradually to reconcile theory-based goals and empirically determined actual performance profiles. This can be achieved by progressively building a consensus in expert groups. While in the earlier case-group approach, the basic methodological problems described could only be inadequately resolved, a new approach to case-group specification has been taken in a new project supported by the German Pensions Insurance and the Federal Ministry for Education and Research in the context of priority support for rehabilitation. The project is planned, in the next two years, to introduce Rehabilitation-Management-Categories (RMK) on a pilot basis for cardiology and orthopedics. The concept of RMK was chosen, firstly because it was conceptually close to the case-groups approach, and secondly, to bring in a central methodology for quality and management concepts.[10]

The RMK, unlike previous approaches, should include both empirically justified clinically relevant rehabilitation case-groups, and theoretical diagnostic and performance-related quality standards reached by consensus. They extend the previously more or less exclusively diagnosis-related definition of case-groups to reflect performance corridors with defined quality requirements. The RMK are envisaged as effective quality management tools through the inclusion of qualitative parameters in the definition of performance. Quality here is concrete in that it starts from the abstract demand for "the best for the patient." It maintains far-reaching practical and strategic dimensions, in that it becomes a direct and immediate component of the definition of performance. If one starts from the basis that this performance target based on the methodical structural principles described is both empirical and theoretical, then the RMK offer an effective form of target treatment standards. They are intended not only to manage performance and quality within the rehabilitation system, but over and above that to be effective within the borderline areas between pre and post treatment care units, i.e., cure and prevention. The RMK develop these integrating functions at no cost and to some extent automatically, in that they pre-define and manage quality. They can thus replace structural measures and post-facto controls and sanctions to ensure quality through the legislator or the rehabilitation provider, which always involves losses.

The integrational function of RMK works through mechanisms such as the following. RMKs focus on quality management relating to the quality of the structure, the process and the outcome. This form of quality management ultimately strengthens the self-reliance and decision-making powers of clinics, not least in relation to the realization of a comprehensive and interdisciplinary approach to treatment, which takes into account both the borders with acute medicine and the after care activities. The effectiveness of this function depends not least on the quality of the target standards or the guidelines themselves. It therefore follows that the inclusion of integrational measures in the definition of quality and performance should be made compulsory, thus making actual performance empirically comparable.

The RMKs underpin the integration of various stages of care and institutions, both in direct patient care as well as in overall institutional planning and management. In relation to patient care, the RMK requires individual management, where the patient under rehabilitation can be "welded" into the whole care system through patient-centered process management based on specific symptoms, therapy and outcome. Centrally, they are an effective tool for network-management, especially important for the management of care structures by rehabilitation institutions and rehabilitation providers within the rehabilitation system and in care units on either side of the demarcation lines. The RMKs support these functions and thus allow them to provide quality and flexible planning of rehabilitation provision and care structures. They also provide the possibility for rehabilitation units to manage their own care performance in a flexible and competitive way, in which integrational measures are effective as a compulsory component of the performance definition as well as having a formative effect.

An important basis for the development of the impact of the RMK lies in information management. Thanks to better documentation of performance, the external and internal transparency of the processes and outcomes is beginning to improve in the clinics. This, however, is a basic precondition for optimizing the structures, processes and outcomes through effective organizational mechanisms in the broadest sense. Not least, the basis of effective financial management has been established through the RMK. This relates not only to the economic relevance of RMK, but also the level of qualitative effects through quality and economic incentives for clinics and all those involved.

Empirical Results from Cardiac Rehabilitation: A Scientific Approach to the Problem of Integration of Acute Medicine, Rehabilitation, and Prevention

Effects of a Changed Curative Treatment Paradigm on Cardiac Rehabilitation

The close interaction of acute medicine, rehabilitation and prevention as an integrated rehabilitative exercise is particularly impressive in the case of cardiology, because this is an area which:

1.   has seen an exceptional effort in recent years especially in acute medicine;

2.   is one of the main causes of death in Germany and thus of special social significance;

3.   is significant as having the second largest demand for inpatient medical rehabilitation;

4.   is relatively well-researched nationally; and not least,

5.   the development of modern rehabilitation in Germany through concepts such as CCC (comprehensive cardiac care) has had a significant influence.

This example should show how changes in acute medical care in the last ten years have affected the profile of cardiac rehabilitation patients and the consequences of that for performance and quality requirements. It is also an example of the empirical inclusion of actual treatment standards in rehabilitation as a starting point for subsequent RMKs and target treatment standards.

The starting point for the research was the development of demand for cardiac rehabilitation in the last ten years against the background of suspicions increasingly expressed in public of growing abuse of social services, which here means the so-called excessive demands on rehabilitation services not sufficiently justified by need.

If one observes the development of demand for cardiac rehabilitation services in insurance for salaried employees in the eight years between 1989 and 1996, there is an astonishing rise of 90 percent (Figure 6.1), in both the old (+47 percent) and the new provinces (+146 percent). In order to ascertain the reasons for this rise, the possible influence of demographic changes was then analyzed. A suitable method for this is age equalization. The result, however, shows that only a small part of the increase can be explained by the demographic ageing of the insured population. Both for the constant age structure 1989-1996 in the old provinces and 1991-1996 for the new, compared with the absolute development, the demand for rehabilitation services is only slightly less for salaried employees. The increase in demand cannot therefore be explained by demographic factors alone.

Another possible cause of the increased demand might be suspected in an increase in the underlying coronary heart disease. The necessary information on the incidence/prevalence of coronary heart disease to ascertain such a relationship appears to be somewhat problematic in several ways in Germany:

1. the indications for cardiac rehabilitation are very broadly drawn (ICD-No. 410-414); and

2. in this context there are no adequate epidemiological data available for the country as a whole. The only data—which are regionalized and confined to a certain form of coronary heart disease with only limited epidemiological value, are based on the results of the MONICA/CORA Study (Löwel et al./Keil et al.).

Against this background a simplified model was selected in which mortality and cause of death were taken as an indicator of cardiac

Figure 6.1
Cardiac Rehabilitation Groups in the BfA

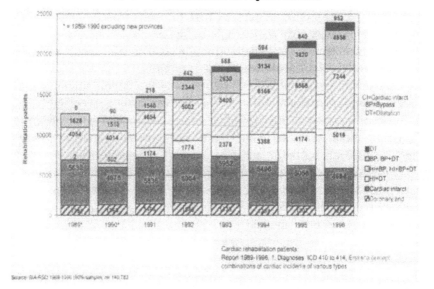

morbidity. The use of mortality as a morbidity indicator relies on the fundamental assumption, adopted in many studies, of a relatively stable ratio of survivors to the total and to deaths from coronary heart disease—in broad terms—with an average for each age-group by study group and region of 50-70 percent.

The second premise, as shown by empirical evidence, has not been demographically verified for the whole population. It has, however, been confirmed by various recent research with random, forecasting and controlled design. The assumption that by new treatment methods, such as the various forms of cardiac intervention and/or ACVB, would bring a fall in deaths or complications in coronary heart disease, especially myocardial infarcts, could not be confirmed. As these results, at least in the Anglo-Saxon world, have been repeated in numerous large-scale analyses (Pocock et al./Sim et al.), the assumption of a relative persistence of death from coronary heart disease and its related incidence and prevalence can be regarded as very likely.

Thus, if one observes the development of mortality from cardiac illnesses in recent years for the population as a whole, an ever increasing trend can be seen (Federal Statistical Office). The analysis resulted in no connection between the ratio of morbidity indicators to mortality ICD-Nr.410-414, and the demand for rehabilitation. It can thus be concluded that the increased demand for rehabilitation cannot have been caused by an increased incidence and prevalence.

In seeking other possible causes for the increased demand, the quest turned to the care provision closely related to rehabilitation. That particularly included patients with myocardial infarcts and related ACVB/PTCA with exclusively conservative treatment and similar patients who, without suffering a myocardial infarcts, underwent bypass operations or cardiac surgery. The reference statistics from the curative provision show hospital cases with and without surgical operations and bypass, such as PTCA cases, which were published by Bruckenberger in a yearly updated report. The growing demand for rehabilitation correlates significantly with the equally strong growth in heart operations and cardiac surgery. The link between coronary patients who have undergone surgery and the increased demand for rehabilitation is also reflected, according to the differentiated pre-treatment, in the indications spectrum of cardiac rehabilitation patients. While in the early 1980s, by far the greatest number of patients in cardiac rehabilitation had been exclusively treated conservatively,[11] in 1996 there was a predominance of coronary patients in rehabilitation who had been operated on or subject to cardiac surgery (Table 6.1). If one starts from the suspicion that there is fundamentally no difference in the pattern of demand related to cardiac infarcts and other coronary illness, one comes to the conclusion that the increase in coronary demand, which is mainly shown by the disproportionate increase in coronary patients undergoing cardiac surgery, is linked to changes in the curative treatment paradigm towards an increase in operative and interventionist methods.

The published results are doubly significant in supporting the need for (cardiac) rehabilitation. Firstly, an external factor in the provision of treatment in acute hospital medicine was examined, whose influence on the demand for rehabilitation, and this concerns primarily the studies into under/over demand for rehabilitation, was previously hardly noticed in quantitative terms. Secondly, the investigative approach also includes qualitative parameters of the patient structure and thus opens the way to internal investigation into external influences, such as the effects of changes in cure on the quality of rehabilitation.

The consideration of differentiated qualitative parameters, however, raises many more unsolved methodological problems, especially relating to performance specification. The search for treatment standards with empirically and theoretically assured qualitative performance profiles sets new challenges to research into rehabilitation, in order to establish epidemiological, and conceptually based modern models, i.e., also capable of forecasting.

Actual Treatment Standards in Cardiac Rehabilitation—the Empirical Basis for RMKs

A first step in this direction was the empirical research into *actual treatment standards* in cardiac rehabilitation, which could establish the basis of subsequent elaboration of target standards. Standards are understood as "standardized values of validated indicators of the quality of structures, processes and outcomes" [Association of Scientific Medical Societies (AWMF), 1995]. Actual standards describe the present, empirically determined range of variations. They set out the so-called "implicit treatment standards." The analysis of actual treatment standards then sets out to achieve transparency and highlight quality as well as quality differences in the treatment (Badura, Grande et al., 1995). The repeated observation of medical measures and their success provides experience of the effectiveness of medical procedures. This empirical knowledge flows continually into the quality of medical rehabilitation, so that in practice it creates so-called implicit standards (Selbmann, 1984; Senftleben, 1980; Winter, 1997). These were studied in relation to cardiac rehabilitation. The starting point was the distinction between the effect on needs of the coronary groups which had been subject to surgery and those that had been treated conservatively. This group was chosen to investigate the effects of changed demand profiles on performance specifications. Based on earlier studies, there was a real suspicion that these groups differed greatly in essential therapy-related characteristics, such as somatic results, psychic and social aspects and the treatment of the illness and the related outcome.

The methodological basis of the analysis was the documentation of cardiac rehabilitation provision according to the so-called therapeutic performance classification. This involves a general classification of indications of rehabilitation cases by type, number, duration and frequency, to include the minimum requirements for therapeutic procedures in terms of quality treatments. This classification system is itself the result of comprehensive empirical analysis of rehabilitation provision and its concluding consensual elaboration based on the theoretical aspects. It also serves as a first step in the direction of quality standardization taking account of wide empirical experience in practice.

The analysis of performance data for the year 1997 for rehabilitation clinics showed that coronary patients in rehabilitation received an average of 65 treatments, with variations as expected between clinics, with a significant emphasis on sport and physical therapy, followed by information services (Figure 6.2).

Further analysis distinguishing between conservatively treated (only cardiac infarct) and surgically (bypass) treated rehabilitation patients shows significant differences. Patients with by-pass operations received less stamina training than those under rehabilitation from heart attacks. In weight training and so-called passive procedures, such as electro, hydro and bathing therapy and massage, the ratio was reversed. Those who had been operated on received less psycho-therapeutic or counseling support, i.e., those aimed at long-term changes in behavior and lifestyle (Figure 6.3).

The interpretation of these empirical results is still awaited. Expert groups will have to explain which empirical findings support the theoretical standards and which can be taken as suggesting a modified approach to the typical classifications of treatment. On this basis RMKs should then be constructed, with a qualitative and quantitative performance specification which can be seen as a step in the direction of ideal treatment standards.

Qualitative Empirical Analyses of Cardiac Rehabilitation—an Example of the Scientific Basis of an Effective Integrated Quality Management

In summary, it can be concluded from the empirical results about the interaction of cardiac acute treatment and rehabilitation under the central theme of integration of prevention, cure and rehabilitation, that they are significant in two ways. Although the study is confined in explicit terms to the area of responsibility of one insurer, the Salaried Employees' Insurance Institution, and one application, cardiac rehabilitation, general external factors in another area of treatment, acute medicine, are analyzed qualitatively at the same time.

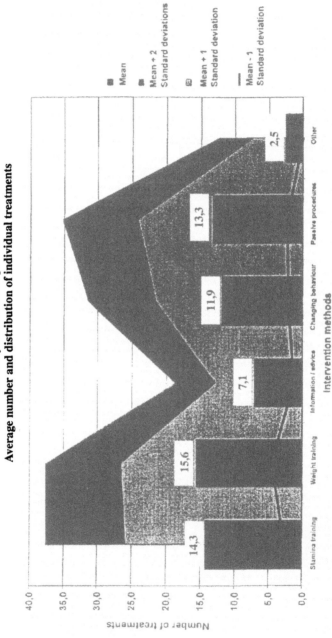

Figure 6.2
Treatment Standards by Method of Intervention
1997 - Coronary heart disease patients overall
Average number and distribution of individual treatments

N = 2.325 (ICD 410-414; Erstreha, AHB, <75 years; in-patient; reg. discharge, duration 18-31 days; clinics with PL-rank 1-15)

Source: BfA, Report 1997.

Figure 6.3
Treatment Profile by Method of Intervention
Actual treatment standards in coronary heart disease rehabilitation - 1997 - by cardiac patient groups

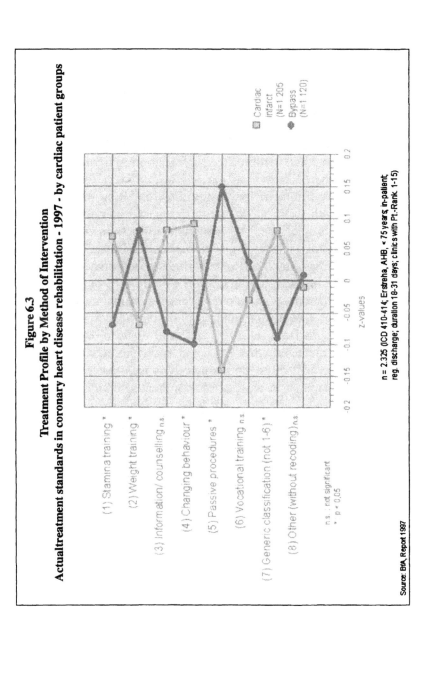

(1) Stamina training *

(2) Weight training *

(3) Information / counselling n.s

(4) Changing behaviour *

(5) Passive procedures *

(6) Vocational training n.s

(7) Generic classification (not 1-6) *

(8) Other (without recoding) n.s

n.s. : not significant
* : p < 0,05

Cardiac infarct (N=1 205)

Bypass (N=1 120)

z-values

-0.2 -0.15 -0.1 -0.05 0 0.05 0.1 0.15 0.2

n = 2.325 (ICD 410-414; Erstreha, AHB, < 75 years; in-patient;
reg. discharge; duration 18-31 days; clinics with Pt.-Rank 1-15)

Source: BfA, Report 1997

This qualitative approach goes beyond the widely used quantitative models, which were especially predominant in estimating need. It allows the qualitative dimensions derived from the analysis to be included in planning and management, and then in an insurer's area of responsibility. On the one hand this relates to the predominant functions of health care in the rehabilitation system and on the other, the process and outcome-oriented differentiation of further quality management functions within the rehabilitation system.

First, *the general aspects of the rehabilitation system*: it is precisely under conditions of increasing differentiation of care structures in the health sector alongside to the growth in networking that it is important to understand the structural impacts more thoroughly in order to minimize demarcation problems and losses. This means, among other things, linking responsibilities based on sectoral structuring for planning and administration of care in a defined area— such as rehabilitation—with an overall extra-systemic oversight. This requirement was recently of fundamental significance in the social policy debate both from the organizational angle of care (patient-centered care, managed care, etc.) and from the economic aspect (cost transfer to cost of economizing). It is true that responsibility for structural planning in an area of treatment is divided operationally between various providers, but it is, nevertheless, part of a general responsibility perceived by society and a global strategy for health care as a whole.

Returning to the problem posed initially of a health insurance scheme not driven purely by market forces, the cardiac rehabilitation model clearly shows that demand is based on supply. In concrete terms, increased availability of alternative cardiac treatments leads to a rise in the number of patients being treated resulting in an increased demand for rehabilitation. The extent to which this development corresponds to social value systems and resources will ultimately be governed by society. In this context, models for requirements can and should take into account both structural changes-- within the rehabilitation system (such as changes in forms of provision) and the boundaries between prior and subsequent areas of treatment.

On the other hand, the rehabilitation system's reflection of the scale of external management also influences the *internal management of rehabilitation systems*. Thus the identification of changed rehabilitation requirements, such as shown in cardiology, leads to corresponding qualitatively differentiated planning and management models relating not only to the structures but also the processes and results of rehabilitation. In specific terms, this means, for example, that for rehabilitation patient groups different forms of rehabilitative therapy can be distinguished, based on need. At this stage scientific rehabilitation models no longer involve superficial quantity management processes, but significant far-reaching issues of process and outcome-oriented quality management. Taking account of qualitatively differentiated parameters thus raises serious questions of scientific rehabilitation research, as yet partly unanswered.

Summary

The integration of prevention, cure and rehabilitation throws up a number of problems in Germany, not least because of the division of responsibility between various providers under social legislation. Quality of care is seen as a prime criteria for strategies to solve the demarcation problem. If quality is central to the management of all processes, so are structural decisions. The precondition for this central function of quality is, however, its translation into effective programs. Here there is still at present a serious need for scientific research. Above all, effective target standards must be developed. They can for the time being be confined to the current comprehensible legally regulated areas of responsibility and delivery, but the demarcation areas should be defined thematically. A significant basis for this development is seen as the definition of patient treatment groups. In rehabilitation, research projects are currently in progress into the development of RMKs. It can thus logically be concluded (to overcome the serious structural deficiencies of other approaches) that RMKs should only be defined by the iterative consensual process of reconciling empirical findings with theory-driven performance demands. In the first stage, existing treatment standards must be included. Empirical results from cardiology are proposed as examples in this connection. They are of particular interest, because here the qualitative effects of changes in the curative treatment paradigm on the quality of cardiac rehabilitation are clear. In a further stage of development, target standards should be introduced as a component of RMKs based on the empirically derived existing standards. The RMKs are seen as a suitable instrument for planning and management of both within rehabilitation systems and external processes. They thus point the way to a methodical approach to the integration of prevention, cure and rehabilitation.

Notes

1. World Health Organization, Regional Office for Europe (Ed.). Glossary of health care technology, *Public Health in Europe* 4; Copenhagen 1975, p. 302.
2. Association of German Pensions Institutions/Rehabilitation-Commission (Ed.): Bd. I-VII, Final report of the Commission for the Development of Rehabilitation in Statutory Pensions Insurance, Frankfurt/M.1991.
3. Council of Experts for Concerted Action in the Health System, special reports 1995, Baden-Baden 1995.
4. Hofmann, E., Agenda item "Rehabilitation—Development of a New Concept," in *German Medical Journal* 96, Vol. 24, 1999, p. C-1158.
5. Müller-Fahrnow, W., Schliehe, F., Spyra, K., The Rehabilitation System with special emphasis on the changing economic conditions, in Bengel, J.; Koch, U. (Ed.) Fundamentals of the Science of Rehabilitation, Springer-Verlag, publication pending.
6. Arrow, K. J., "Uncertainty and the Welfare Economics of Medical Care, Collected Papers," *Applied Economics*, Vol. 6. London 1985, pp. 15-50.
7. "Outcomes and PORTs," in *The Lancet*, Vol. 340: 12 December1992, 1439.
8. Leitlinien-In-Fo, the guidelines information and further education program of the Medical Centre for Quality Assurance, in documents of the Medical Centre for Quality Assurance, Vol. 1; Bern, Vienna, New York, 1998, p.3.
9. Mansky, Th., Case-group systems, in F & W 3/97, 14th Year, p. 210 et seq.
10. Spyra, K., Müller-Fahrnow, W., "Rehabilitation-Management-Categories (RMK)—a new approach to the structuring of case-groups in medical rehabilitation," in *Rehabilitation* 37, Suppl.1 (1998), 47-56.
11. Müller-Fahrnow, W., "A critical social and epidemiological approach to the system of medical rehabilitation," in *Deutsche Hochschulschriften* 2557; Hänsel Hohenhausen; Egelsbach, Frankfurt a. M., Washington, 1998.

7

New Benefits Dealing with Ageing Populations: Long-Term Care

X. Scheil-Adlung

There is increasing concern in many countries that social security in the area of long-term care is in serious deficiencies: costs are rising uncontrollably, there are not enough beds in residential care homes and arrangements for care at home are non-existent or quite inadequate. Moreover, it is likely that given the global ageing of the population, the demand for care of the elderly will increase further in the future.

That is why in many OECD countries in recent years, reforms of social insurance and dependency have been discussed and to some extent introduced. The starting point for new approaches to care policies in most countries is controlling costs in the health systems, which seek to limit the use of high cost care. At the same time, conceptual and administrative issues have been raised, which require old-age provision to be coordinated with other areas of social security.

Which concepts and strategies are regarded as able to control the growing care needs through the health system, other social security systems or private provision? What should be the goals of the new care policies? How can they be achieved through new forms of organization, financing methods and services? What are the core political issues that need to be clarified through the introduction of new benefits and regulations on care?

The following chapter addresses these issues. First the causes of the worldwide increase in demand for care will be investigated, with emphasis on the demographic and socioeconomic context. Next, new political ideas and strategies to overcome the problems of care provision will be explored and illustrated taking the example of Germany's care provision.

Causes of the Rising Demand for Care

A comparison between the population indicators for 1950 and 1998 in most countries shows a shift from high mortality and birth rates to lower mortality and birth rates.[1] This shift, frequently described as the ageing of the population, is faster in the industrialized countries than in developing countries and is the most discussed demographic trend of the twenty-first century.

Greater life expectancy and falling birth rates mean not only that the absolute number of old people is rising, but also that the over-65 age group, especially people who survive past 80, is growing faster than other age groups. Thus, if past trends continue, the majority of old people will be women, as women's life expectancy worldwide is higher than men's.

A comparison of the life expectancy of men and women in 1950 and 1998 in selected regions of the world can be found in Table 7.1.

The table shows clearly that life expectancy in the observation period of 48 years in all the developing and industrialized countries examined has risen, sometimes dramatically, as in China by 28.8 years (women), sometimes less markedly, as in the USA by only 6.9 years (men).

It is also clear that the highly industrialized countries of Asia and Europe have the oldest population, while the youngest population is in Africa. The pace of ageing appears most pronounced in developing countries, especially Asia.

Equally significant for the future development of health systems and care provision is, however, not only demographic ageing as such but also the extent to which increasing age is linked to impaired health and the extent to which traditional carers (daughters, wives) remain available.

New research[2] shows that the extra years of life gained by old people are largely without an increase in impairment of health. Thus, 65-year-old men in Switzerland can expect to live 70 percent of their remaining years without any disability. For women, the percentage is some 76 percent.

Table 7.1
Life Expectancy at Birth in Selected Countries, 1950 and 1998

Region/country	Men		Women	
	1950	1998	1950	1998
Africa				
Egypt	41.2	60.1	43.6	64.1
Ghana	40.4	54.8	43.6	58.9
South Africa	44.0	53.6	46.0	57.8
America				
USA	66.0	72.9	71.7	79.6
Argentina	60.4	70.9	65.1	78.3
Costa Rica	56.0	73.5	58.6	78.5
Mexico	49.2	68.6	52.4	74.8
Asia				
Australia	66.7	77.0	71.8	83.0
Japan	59.6	76.9	63.1	83.3
China	39.3	68.3	42.3	71.1
Europe				
Germany	64.6	73.8	68.5	80.3
Denmark	68.9	73.6	71.5	79.1
France	63.7	74.6	69.4	82.6
Greece	63.4	75.8	66.7	81.0
Austria	62.0	74.1	67.0	80.7
Sweden	69.9	76.5	72.6	82.0
Hungary	59.3	66.5	63.4	75.4

Source: U.S. Census Bureau, International Brief: Gender and Aging, Washington, October 1998.

Only in Australia can women expect to live a greater part of their remaining life without disability than men. In the other countries, women must expect to need care earlier than men.

Alongside great age, its rapid rise and the feminization of the elderly population, a characteristic of the group of (potential) dependents in developing and industrialized countries is the increasing decline in the care capacity of family members. This trend is due to:

Figure 7.1
Diability-free years of life after age 65 as a percentage, 1991

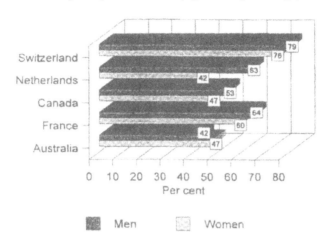

Source: J. Robine; I. Romieu, loc.cit., 1993.

- fewer children,

- male mortality, and

- more women working.

Correspondingly, an individualization[3], i.e., living in single-person households rather than multigeneration families, can be seen.

The trends described above mean not only that needs for care will rise further in the future, but also that there is a necessity of developing new approaches. Thus, the decline in the care capacity of families should result in the need to seek new formal and informal forms of care. The simultaneous pressure on social security budgets and especially the health system thus calls for special expert and political imagination.

New Political Approaches and Strategies to Long-Term Care of the Elderly

In the past, the predominant feature of care policies in many countries was a proliferation of regulations and arrangements, frequently marked by a lack of coherent national care policies. Despite many

individual laws, only in a few countries was there an integrated solution to problems that can be found in other areas of social security
such as old age, illness, unemployment. In many countries, there
was a general expectation that the care of the elderly infirm was a
family responsibility and later an area for community voluntary undertakings.

This may be due to the fact that dependency in old age must be
regarded as a relatively new risk and, from the social security stand-
point, falls in the gap between the traditional risks of old age, illness,
accident and disability. Depending on the social security system, it
may also involve social services, welfare and private support services. This led to a plethora of regulations and jurisdictions at various administrative levels which made a comprehensive solution to
the problem much more difficult. Only a few countries, for example,
the Netherlands and Israel, had legislated provisions for long-term
care as an amendment to their social security systems, to deal with
these needs of the elderly.

As a result of the constantly rising costs of health provision and
deficiencies in national social welfare regulations, there was an increase of political will to tackle the health-care problem in a systematic way and to undertake a cost effective and political reassessment
of the risks related to care needs.

An international comparison of expenditure on care services as a
percentage of health expenditure in 1994 shows that it ranged from
18 percent in Denmark to 10.4 percent in Belgium[4].

The changes in the period 1980 to 1994 range from an increase
of 6.6 percent in Belgium and a slight fall in expenditure in Denmark, Canada and the Netherlands, as can be seen from Table 7.2
below.

Cost analysis suggests some inappropriate health care provisions,
such as occupation of beds in medical hospitals with long-term care
patients, as special care facilities are either inadequate or non-existent. This means that services are provided by highly qualified health
workers, when the same services—such as help with personal care
to carry out the activities of daily living—could be performed by
less-qualified staff.

To avoid this trend becoming more acute, in recent years several
OECD countries have brought in reforms which have partly led to
comprehensive and coordinated care solutions. Fundamental health

Table 7.2
Care Services as a Percentage of Health Expenditure in Selected Countries

Country	1994	Change 1980-1994
Australia	14	0.9
Belgium	10.4	6.6
Canada	11.9	-0.6
Denmark	18.0	-0.1
Netherlands	13.9	-0.5
United Kingdom	17.2	1.4
USA	11.5	1.4

Source: M. Schneider, loc. cit., p. 158.

Table 7.3
New and Existing Regulations for Long-Term
Care in Selected European Countries

Country	Care provision	Financing	Private alternatives
Austria	Since 1993, cash benefits under various social welfare headings, which can be exchanged for services in kind	Taxation and contributions	Can be paid for using cash benefits
France	For some years, experiments with services in kind and cash benefits	National Budget, social welfare	Limited availability
Germany	Since 1995, social care provision covers home care and institutional care, services in kind and cash benefits	1.7 per cent of income of employees and pensioners	Care provision component
Luxemburg	Since 1998, care provision covered by institutional, formal and informal care, mainly through services in kind, that can be exchanged for cash benefits	45 per cent of expenditure from the National Budget, special contribution by the electricity industry, 1 per cent of total income of insured	
Netherlands	For a long time, covered under the Exceptional Medical Expenses Scheme	Contributions by employers and self-employed	
Norway	Medical and long-term care covered by the existing system	Taxation	Development of private ventures
United Kingdom	Under the National Health Service	Taxation	

Source: Pacolet, J.; Bouten, R.; Lanoye, H.; Versieck, K.: Social protection for dependency in old age in the 15 EU Member States and Norway, Leuven, 1998, and own research.

system reforms were carried out in Europe (Germany, Austria and Luxembourg).5 Other countries, such as the United Kingdom, have introduced or extended targeted help for those in need of care or are now considering doing so, for example, France.

Table 7.3 sets out the basic new regulations and some well-established ones, in selected European countries.

Even some highly industrialized countries in Asia and the Pacific have introduced new regulations on care provision or are considering doing so. Thus, reforms have been carried out in recent years in Australia and New Zealand. In Japan,[6] it is intended to bring in a new comprehensive reform in the year 2000.

Targets of Reform

At the forefront of these solutions there are general targets which also affect other health reforms, especially cost control through the involvement of market elements.[7] In addition, proposed goals

Table 7.4
Leading Care Reform Targets of OECD Countries

Benefits and services
• Enhanced quality of benefits and services provision • Increased efficiency in benefits and service delivery • Priority to outpatient services over inpatient
Financing
• Cost control • Contribution/tax ceilings • Reduced expenditure on health insurance and social welfare
Individuals/insured persons
• Prevention of excessive demands on benefits and services • Prevention of dependence on social welfare • Prevention of excessive costs to individuals • Prevention of poverty
Institutions
• Relief of institutions • Expansion of long-term care infrastructure

specific to care provision can also be found in the reform proposals.

Frequently found reform targets8 for care provision in OECD countries are shown in the following table.

Thus, reforms will be decided and implemented, both in services and expenditure as well as on the individual and institutional level.

The overriding desire of many politicians to relieve the burden on health and social welfare systems is reflected in the following goals: cost control, reduction in the expenditure on health insurance and social welfare, prevention of excessive demands on services, prevention of dependence on social welfare and relief of institutions.

Often several goals are sought simultaneously. Thus the priority given to outpatient rather than inpatient services is linked to the prospect of being able to offer better services, make savings, prevent poverty and reduce the need for residential homes. This can, among other things, be achieved through the provision of informal care by family members, who are often not only the best, but also the cheapest, form of care.

Performance targets such as enhanced quality and efficiency can be attained, for example, by the introduction of quality standards and regular evaluation in the framework of the extension and establishment of formal and informal welfare provision.

The cost burden on individuals can be controlled by caps on contributions and taxes, avoidance of excessive charges to individuals and prevention of poverty.

Forms of Care Organization

How can the stated goals be translated into organizational forms of care provision?

Here we have two alternative possibilities:

- Revision and extension of existing regulations for old age, illness, accident and social welfare, as in Australia, Ireland, New Zealand or Austria.

  In this solution, health and welfare provision is frequently integrated. It is thus also possible for several social welfare departments to be responsible for care provision. Cash benefits can therefore be delivered by other social welfare providers and departments than services.

- Establishment of a new insurance system to cover long-term care within the existing social security scheme, as, for example, in Germany.

This solution, unlike the first, allows the introduction of separate budgets for care and thus better control of costs and use of resources than would be possible under a general administrative framework, for example, health insurance.

With the introduction of a separate insurance method, it will also be possible to introduce new structural elements into social insurance not available in existing branches, which could be useful in long-term care provision. These include:

- A new basis of compulsory or voluntary insured groups of persons, which do not have to coincide with the groups under other branches of social insurance. Thus, for example, the individual's compulsory insurance contribution can be limited for those aged 40 and over.

- The introduction of new forms of insurance in the area of long-term care provision, without changing existing branches of social security, such as the involvement of profit-oriented private insurance into the social security scheme. It is conceivable that compulsory long-term care insurance could be introduced partly or fully through private profit-oriented insurance.

Financing of Social Security for Care Needs

Essentially, "traditional" methods of financing social security were retained in the countries that introduced reforms:

- pay-as-you-go in the framework of social insurance;
- tax-based financing through state programs, such as income-related social welfare.
- In the case of profit-oriented private insurance, the funding approach is used.

The introduction of the above goals in the area of financing creates serious problems for many countries. As the starting point for most reforms in long-term care provision is cost reduction in health care, there is a danger that existing state resources cannot, in the long term be adequate. In particular, because of the grey area between their application to acute medical treatment and long-term care, it is to be feared that resources will be pushed towards expensive medical treatment.

A particular problem is the relationship between the target of reducing the cost burden to the state and preventing greater cost burdens on individuals. These conflicting goals have in most of the reforming countries led to solutions which only partly cover the cost of care through the public purse and build on the increased provision of private resources.

A comprehensive insurance of long-term care, exclusively from public or private resources, is not to be found in the reforming countries. In the context of the reform process, the existing mixed financing by public and private resources has been retained or extended.

The reformists saw "financial room for maneuver" in the income and capital situation of old people. In addition, it is assumed that economic activity at increasing age does not have to be restricted, but can be allowed to continue, unless precluded by early retirement, early-retirement pension rules, etc.

The income and capital situation of old people is not only relevant to the provision of age-related services, which are income-related—such as care provided by the social welfare system.[9] The increasing groups of contributors and taxpayers who finance long-term care provision and provide co-payments are also an aspect of the new care provision arrangements.

Thus, the German and Japanese reform legislation provides for financing of long-term care through contributions by the insured, co-payments, as well as through public subsidies.

Benefit Design

When it comes to benefit design in long-term care provision, similar solutions can be found in the various reform processes. This includes the introduction of the following core innovations in the performance aspect of most reforms:

- Attendance allowances

- New in-kind benefits—including health promotion and early detection of chronic disease

- Social security coverage of carers

Attendance allowances are the most significant innovation concerning long-term care benefits. They are paid to cover the cost of home care and not to replace the beneficiary's income, as is the case with other cash social security benefits.

In most countries, attendance allowances are paid either directly to the persons in need of care or to the carer(s). In the case of direct payments to the persons needing care, this allows the possibility of employing one or more people and making a choice.

They generally consist of flat-rate payments, which individuals must use to cover the services they use. In countries with social insurance schemes, the predominant model is direct payments to those in need without any income-related means testing.

Less frequently, income-related payments are made direct to the carers. This is particularly the case in the Scandinavian countries, where informal carers, such as family members or neighbors, receive lower incomes in the context of communal households.[10]

Basically, there are graded levels of attendance allowances, depending on the degree of care needed, which are linked to the extent of assistance needed in carrying out the activities of daily living and health services which can be provided in the home. The distinction is often based on the following criteria, which may be further subdivided in various countries:

- dependent persons,

- seriously dependent persons,

- totally dependent persons.

Classification in the various categories is often by official doctors or medical services, who in some cases collaborate with the authorities that pay the attendance allowances, and based on medical and functional assessment and needs for health and personal care.

The amount of the home attendance allowance is not only always less than the cost of inpatient care, but also less than the allowances paid for residential care.

Newly developed in-kind benefits are mainly related to the introduction and extension of facilities for home care, based on a combination of professional and informal services, such as personal care by family members.[11] The (partial) assumption of the costs of this service is paid either as an alternative or as a top-up for the attendance allowance. A special concern is thus to achieve a better linkage between outpatient services and residential or semi-residential services.

Prominent here is another new function: support for informal carers who alone or with professional services provide day and night home services such as invalid care, housework, help with dressing, etc.

In order to prepare informal carers for their work and provide them with support, advice to and training of family carers, neighbors and voluntary helpers is increasingly offered as a new service.

A further innovation with regard to benefits can be seen in social protection for carers. Carers are not only often able to take leave from their job, but also during the period of care to acquire and increase their social protection. Social protection for carers is, however, limited to pension and accident insurance.

In some countries, the provision of holiday replacements during the care period is also included in the list of benefits.

In addition to the extension of long-term residential care in special care centers, in many countries there is increased expansion of semi-residential care for those in need. These take various forms of day care centers specially equipped for old people.

Core Issues in the Introduction of New Regulations for Care Provision

Regardless of which solution to insuring against the old-age dependency risk is chosen, there arise the same problem areas and core issues in care reform. These issues relate to the financial and administrative aspects of dependency and lie frequently at the heart of political discussions of reform. They include four problem areas, which will be briefly discussed below:

- the distinction to be made between the need for long-term care and medical health care, i.e., between long-term care and acute medical treatment;

- centralization or decentralization of organization and service provision;

- long-term care insurance through the public and/or private sector;

- development of the infrastructure for the range of long-term care benefits;

Distinction between Long-Term Care and Medical Health Care

It is often observed that a sharper distinction should be made between medical health care, disability and age, in order to allow better management of costs and services in specific programs or branches of social security, for example, long-term care insurance, social assistance, health insurance or pensions insurance. Such a clarification facilitates cost calculations and the establishment of budgets for long-term care provision.

The definition of dependency is confined in many countries to a state requiring support through regular, repeated activities in daily life, such as bodily or "personal" care , feeding and mobility. However, an overlap with health care, especially in the case of chronic or multiple disease, cannot be excluded.

In many countries, therefore, the degree of dependency is assessed by special procedures in each case, in order to restrict access to services to the most dependent. These procedures generally take into account the functional disability of the individual and the stage of disease or disability which causes the dependence.

Centralization or Decentralization of Organization and Service Provision?

The fundamental decision is whether long-term care provision should be organized centrally by the state or decentralized.

The advantages of central provision are certainly equal access by all dependents to services and the avoidance of "service differences" in individual districts. In addition, central or national programs generally involve lower administrative costs than locally managed programs.

The disadvantages of centralization[12] are often seen that the service structures in local care are highly developed and the planning and provision of services must take local conditions into account. The greater flexibility and less bureaucracy of decentralization allow more account to be taken of local values (for example, religious values).

Long-Term Care Provision through the Public or Private Sector?

The question of to what extent insurance and long-term care provision should be provided through the public or private sector is related to rising costs, service quality and the solidarity element (redistribution aspect). Among other things, a distinction can be drawn between the following areas:[13]

- Public or private compulsory or voluntary insurance or provision through a national program financed from taxation (like national health services). This decision will usually establish the coverage of the scheme as well as the basis of its financing (contribution/taxation or private resources).

The Nordic countries decided to include long-term care provision in their national health programs. Other countries with social security schemes chose compulsory insurance as in Germany, which can include private insurance schemes.

- Services can be provided through national or regional administrations, state enterprises, autonomous government bodies, private cooperative bodies, or non-government organizations, private non-profit and for-profit entities.

In the countries concerned, priority is given to decreasing inpatient care in favor of outpatient or ambulatory care. The focus of long-term care is home care, which could also reduce some need for extended stays in general hospitals, as well as in residential institutions.

There could be a problem in this respect due to a lack of a coordinating network of the various service providers between hospital and community services. That could lead to under- or over-supply, administrative duplication and frictional inefficiencies.

- The introduction of competition between public and/or private enterprises plays a central role in the health schemes of OECD countries and is also relevant to long-term care provision. Questions to be answered here are, for example: What is the financial effect of "competition" between informal and formal services, between outpatient and residential care, and how can informal care arrangements or providers meet the required quality standards?

Development of a Care Infrastructure

In many industrialized countries, neither home care nor residential care is sufficiently developed to meet the growing demand. There is an enormous lack of day centers for old people, services such as "meals-on-wheels," personal care and home visits, old-age homes and residential care. In order to allow the development of a care infrastructure, massive investment is often needed to cover needs for physical facilities, equipment and training. These elements therefore have to be included in the national, regional and local health services planning efforts.

Case Study: Social Long-Term Care Insurance in Germany

It is frequently sought to provide long-term care insurance in the framework of a national social and political philosophy. So, too, in Germany, as well as in other countries with social insurance schemes, it was sought to provide dependency insurance in the context of social insurance. By way of example, the new regulations on dependency insurance introduced in Germany in 1995 are described below.

Organizational Arrangements

In Germany the social long-term care insurance was established as a separate insurance scheme to supplement the statutory insurance system for old age, health care, accident and unemployment.

Care services are provided to the insured person and family members. These services should serve to maintain or restore dependents' activity. Outpatient medical rehabilitation services can also be brought in. The quality of the services should meet generally accepted standards of medical care.

Long-term care insurance providers are administered by the statutory health insurance. These are independent public corporations.

The coverage of long-term care insurance equals the coverage of the statutory health insurance. This is some 90 percent of the population. The remainder of the population must insure themselves privately, through private health insurance.

Financing

Expenditure on long-term insurance is currently around DM 31 billion. It is financed through contributions by the insured. The amount is currently 1.7 percent of monthly salary. The amount is paid half by the employer and half by the employee.

In Germany, further innovative ways of providing resources have been explored to find new sources of financing. In addition to the normal contribution-based financing by employers and employees, State supplements were introduced, for example, to invest in residential care, and a statutory holiday was abolished. That would partly compensate the employer for the burden of the dependency insurance contribution.

A further innovation in the financing of German long-term care insurance is that coverage of deficits by the State would be terminated. Thus, any excess expenditure by the dependency insurance must in the long term be covered by contribution income.

This decision meant that the long-term care insurance otherwise financed by transfer from the normal fluctuation reserve also retains financial surpluses to cover demographic risks. The surplus on statutory long-term care insurance at the end of 1998 was DM 9.5 billion.[14] With the introduction of long-term care insurance, the burden on social assistance, especially for "care support" services, fell by some DM 8 billion between 1995 and 1996.[15]

Provision of Service and Benefit

At present, some 1.5 million people benefit from/or receive long-term care insurance services in Germany. The costs of these services are not, however, always fully covered and must be supplemented by resources from other social protection schemes, such as social assistance, or from the insured's own resources.

When long-term care services are requested, the long-term care insurance arranges for the health insurance medical service to check whether the conditions for long-term care are met and what scope and level of care is needed. The health insurance medical service consists of some 2,000 doctors and 700 care specialists nationwide who are responsible for the assessments.

The degree of dependency and the medical condition determine the benefits and services provided. Category I comprises people who need help with bodily care, feeding or mobility at least once a day (one and a half hours) and help with housework several times a week.

Seriously dependent people come into category II. The care requirement is at least three times a day (three hours) and several times a week for help with housework.

Category III is where care is required day and night (at least five hours a day) and help with housework several times a week.

The following types of service for old people must be distinguished:[16]

Home care: in this area a distinction should be made between services in kind, cash benefits, combined in-kind and cash benefits, home care in the absence of regular carers, equipment and technical aids, social security coverage for the carer and long-term care training.

- Services in kind

  Home care by professional carers covers all household services and basic personal services such as washing, help with dressing, etc. These benefits can be claimed up to DM 750 for category I, up to DM 1,800 for category II, up to DM 2,800 for category III and hardship cases up to DM 3,750. Costs in excess of these levels must be paid privately.

- Cash benefits

  If the care is provided by an alternative means, for example, spouse, neighbour, etc., the amount of cash benefit for category I is DM 400, for category II DM 800 and for category III DM 1,300.

- Combined cash and in-kind benefits

  Cash and in-kind benefits can be combined; for example, if the service amount is only partly used, then the insured receives a partial cash benefit in addition, according to the dependency category.

- Home care in the absence of regular carers

  Dependents who received cash benefits to pay for home care are also entitled to payment for a substitute home help for up to four weeks a year. A maximum of DM 2,800 is allowed for this. The substitute help is for the period of the carer's holiday or illness, for example.

- Equipment and technical aids

  Long-term care insurance also covers aids such as wheelchairs and financial subsidies are available for adapting the home, provided that this is needed on the grounds of long-term dependency and not sickness. The total amount is DM 60 per month for the use of equipment and up to DM 5,000 for home modifications. Technical aids should normally be acquired through loan arrangements.

- Social security for the carer

  Long-term care insurance covers the informal carer's pension contributions. If the carer returns to regular work, the carer can claim a so-called remuneration grant from the unemployment insurance. Accidents related to care are covered by the accident insurance.

- Care training for family members and voluntary carers

  In order to lighten the mental and physical burden of care for informal carers, free training and courses are available.

Semi-residential care services include day and night care and short-term care.

- Day and night care

  Semi-residential care offers special day and night care in special centers as well as return transport. Services in centers are provided up to the value of DM 750 for category I, up to DM 1,500 for category II and up to DM 2,100 per month for category III.

- Short-term care

  Where home care cannot be provided temporarily, short-term care can be provided in residential centers. This is possible for up to four weeks a year, with an entitlement up to DM 2,800.

Fully residential care services in centers are paid up to DM 2,800 per month and in hardship cases up to DM 3,300. However, this amount may not exceed 75 percent of the center's charges. In total, the average annual cost of dependents under the dependency insurance should not exceed DM 30,000.

Conclusions

The problem of long-term dependency arises in almost all countries, particularly with the ageing of the populations. Yet only a few social security schemes are equipped to deal with it.

Since the early 1990s, significant reforms have been carried out in countries with social insurance systems. Thus, comprehensive new regulations were introduced in Austria in 1993, Germany in 1994, France in 1995 and Luxemburg in 1998. Japan likewise envisages a far-reaching reorganization of long-term care provision in the form of social insurance.

In the context of these reforms, the following new socio-political developments stand out:

- Long-term care services are seen as a new risk and are either:
    - incorporated into the social system as a separate branch of insurance, or
    - built on to the existing sickness, pensions, accident and social welfare system.
- New forms of financing long-term care services include, inter alia:
    - the abolition of statutory holidays,
    - greater co-payment and partial coverage of the cost of the service claimed,
    - introduction of informally provided services.
- Lump-sum home care services include:
    - cash benefits covering part of the formal and informal help,
    - new opportunities for short-term semi-residential care,
    - introduction of social security coverage and training for family carers.
- Integrated cooperation in service delivery between:
    - health care, old age and accident, social assistance and social services,
    - public and private sector.

The former strategy of providing care for the elderly through family members or on a community voluntary basis appears in the longer term not sustainable in many countries. Not only because of demographic trends, but also because of the pressure of ever-rising costs of health insurance and social assistance systems, it can be expected that the number of countries providing dependency insurance as part of the social security system will increase further in the future.

Notes

1. Wojtzak, A. 1998. "Ageing of the world: A challenge to health systems in the 21st century," in: *Delegate Handbook*, Third Annual Summit in International Managed Care Trends, Miami.
2. Robine, J.-M.; Romieu, I. 1993. *Statistical World Yearbook on Health Expectancy*, Laboratoire d'Epidémiologie et d'Economie de la Santé, Montpellier.
3. Bureau of the Census, "An Aging World, II," *International Population Reports*, Washington, 1992, p.52 et seq.
4. Schneider, M. 1998. "Gesundheitssysteme im internationalen Vergleich," Übersichten 1997, Augsburg, p.158.
5. Scheil-Adlung, X. 1995. "Social security for dependent persons in Germany and other countries: Between tradition and innovation," in *International Social Security Review*, 1, p.19 et seq.
6. Schulte, B. 1998. Probleme der Pflegefallabsicherung—Vergleichendes Referat, anläßlich des Deutsch-Japanischen Colloquiums "Probleme der Kranken- und Pflegeversicherung, Rottach-Egern, May, p.7 et seq., unpublished manuscript.
7. Scheil-Adlung:, X. 1999. "Schlaglicht auf international bedeutende Gesundheitsreformen der letzten Jahre" in: *Soziale Sicherheit*, 1, P.45 et seq.
8. Based on Rothgang, H. 1997. "Die Wirkungen der Pflegeversicherung," in *Archiv für Wissenschaft und Praxis der sozialen Arbeit*, 3, p.192.
9. Schulte, B. 1998. Probleme der Pflegefallabsicherung—Vergleichendes Referat, anläßlich des Deutsch-Japanischen Colloquiums "Probleme der Kranken- und Pflegeversicherung, Rottach-Egern, May, p.7 et seq., unpublished manuscript.
10. Schunk, M. 1998. Antworten auf das Pflegedilemma: Pflegepolitische Maßnahmen, Zielsetzungen und Inhalte im Vergleich" in *Internationale Vereinigung für Soziale Sicherheit, Entwicklungen und Tendenzen in der sozialen Sicherheit*, 26. Generalversammlung, Marrakesch, 25.-31. Oktober, unpublished.
11. Schunk, M. 1998. Antworten auf das Pflegedilemma: Pflegepolitische Maßnahmen, Zielsetzungen und Inhalte im Vergleich" in Internationale Vereinigung für Soziale Sicherheit, Entwicklungen und Tendenzen in der sozialen Sicherheit, 26. Generalversammlung, Marrakesch, 25.-31. Oktober, unpublished.
12. Wojtzak, A. 1998. "Ageing of the world: A challenge to health system in 21st century," in *Delegate Handbook*, Third Annual Summit in International Managed Care Trends, Miami.
13. Saltman, R. 1998. "Angebot an Gesundheitsleistungen: Auf dem Weg zu einer Teilung der Aufgaben zwischen dem öffentlichen und privaten Sektor? Die angemessene Rolle des öffentlichen Sektors im Vergleich zum privaten bei der Finanzierung von Gesundheitsleistungen," in *Internationale Vereinigung für Soziale Sicherheit*, Berichte der Technischen Konferenzen der IVSS aus dem Dreijahreszeitraum 1996-1998, Harmonisierung ökonomischer Entwicklungen und

sozialer Bedürfnisse, 26. Generalversammlung, Marrakesch, 25-31. Oktober, unpublished.
14.   Kaula, K. 1999. Die soziale Pflegeversicherung in Deutschland, manuscript of the report on the AIM symposium on 26 March in Barcelona.
15.   "Kurznachrichten für den eiligen Leser," in *Wege zur Sozialversicherung*, Vol. 3, 53rd year, March 1999, p. 93.
16.   The following extracts are taken from the 1.1.1999 version of the Sozialgesetzbuch (Social Legislative Code) (SGB IX).

8

Establishment of Long-Term
Care Insurance Scheme in Japan

N. Iguchi

Japan's new long-term care insurance scheme will begin in the spring of 2000. The new scheme is unique in that all benefits will be provided in kind. By way of comparison, in Germany, where there is a free choice between cash and in-kind benefits, most benefits take the form of cash.

Prior to drafting the new Law, representatives of various fields participated in discussions on how to establish the scheme. This chapter explains the new scheme as a whole and is intended to share our experiences of its legislative process.

Background

It was about fifty years ago that rapid demographic change became evident in Japan. Over a very long period, probably more than 1,000 years, the average life expectancy had been 50 years at the most.

However, the age structure dramatically changed after the Second World War, mainly because of a lower mortality rate, particularly in infants, and greater life expectancy. These have been underpinned by consistent and rapid economic growth. As a result, the proportion of total population made up by older people (aged 65 and over) advanced to over 15 percent in 1998 and is forecast to rise much more rapidly in the very near future. By the same token, the number of older people who are bedridden, senile or frail has drastically increased.

Figure 8.1
Population Pyramids in 1920, 1990, and 2025

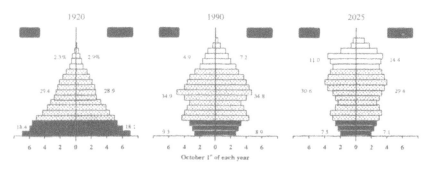

Source: "1995 Population Census of Japan," Statistics Bureau, Managment and Cordination Agency; "Future Population Projection for Japan, estimated in January 1997 (Medium Projection)," National Institute of Population and Social Security Research.

Japan's rapid economic growth and the modernization of its social and family structures have influenced changes to the traditional ways of supporting older family members. This is especially so in the rural areas, where agriculture had long been the dominant industry; younger people have moved out to the urban areas for better job opportunities, leaving their parents behind. Accordingly, social services have been needed to replace traditional family support. In the urban areas, the same kinds of needs have emerged because sons or daughters who are themselves elderly are unable to help their aged parents, particularly those who are bedridden, senile or frail.

The government has been taking the necessary steps to deal with these situations by establishing the Welfare Law for the Elderly, which offers grants to local governments or other organizations concerned with providing services for older people. Largely owing to financial restrictions, these traditional services mainly focus on aid for low-income older people and have not necessarily reached the elderly population as a whole.

This has led the government to consider alternative provisions to meet the need for vast new personal social services for older people. In 1996, the government decided to establish a new long-term care insurance scheme and submitted a bill to Parliament. The bill passed in December 1997, with implementation to begin in the spring of 2000.

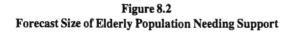

Figure 8.2
Forecast Size of Elderly Population Needing Support

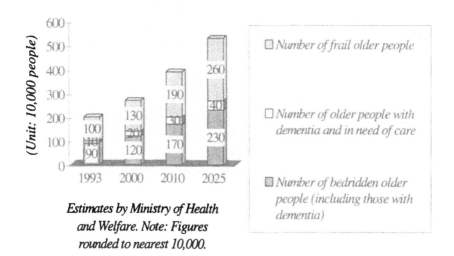

Estimates by Ministry of Health
and Welfare. Note: Figures
rounded to nearest 10,000.

Current Health and Welfare System for Older People in Japan

In the current system, health and medical services for older people are assured under the Health and Medical Service Law for the Aged, established in 1982, while welfare services come under the Welfare Law for the Elderly, established in 1963.

Health and Medical Services for Older People

Older people aged over 70 (and those between 65 and 69 with a disability) qualify for medical services, such as doctor and hospital services, by paying a very limited portion of the costs. In 1999, in the case of outpatient care, older people have to pay only 530 yen for each visit and a portion of prescribed medicine costs (payment is limited to a maximum 2,120 yen a month), while inpatient care costs 1,200 yen a day plus payment for canteen services (in July 1999, US\$ 1 = 121 yen approx.).

Medical costs are financed by contributions from all insurers of the health insurance schemes in addition to central and local government grants. As medical costs for older people have soared, reaching over one-third of total costs, insurance organizations have raised their voices against an increase in insurer contributions.

In response, the government has set up a new advisory council to review the current system.

With the aid of the grant from central government, local governments have provided preventive health services, such as periodic health checks, to prevent disease and promote older people's health.

Welfare Services for Older People

Current welfare services can be divided into facility services and non-facility services. These services are provided either by certain non-profit organizations empowered to act on behalf of the local government or by the local government itself.

Facility services include special nursing homes for older people, care homes, live-in welfare centers for older people and some other facilities. Three-fourths of the construction costs for special nursing homes and all the running costs are financed by central and local governments, which also partly finance other facilities. Non-facility services include home help, short-stay services, day services and other miscellaneous services. Providers of non-facility services can also expect a grant from the government.

Recipients of these facility or non-facility services pay a fee in accordance with an income scale based on criteria established by the government. In reality, most elderly beneficiaries do not pay for their care, or pay a very limited amount if they do. This is because the income scale was set commensurate with beneficiaries' income and thus favors those on low incomes.

Preparatory Discussions about the New Scheme

Those with an interest in the new scheme, such as representatives of local governments, medical associations, welfare service providers, labor unions, employers' organizations and academic groups took part in the discussions about drafting the bill. The debate centered on the following four points: (1) financial resources, (2) choice of insurer, (3) coverage, and (4) benefits.

Financial Resources: Insurance or Public Service

The new scheme is insurance-based (see detailed discussion below), but some insisted that an insurance system for older people could not work well, because the base needed for its introduction was lacking. In other words, since older people are subject to a much higher risk of illness than other population groups, it is almost impossible to set up an insurance system specifically to cover them.

Those holding this view maintained that long-term care services for older people should be funded through taxation instead of insurance contributions. However, most people were in favor of an insurance system because the social insurance system has more impression on people of right to benefits than taxation does and the cost-and-benefit concept is more evident in the social insurance system than in taxation.

The insurer: Central Government or Local Government

The new insurance scheme is to be run by the basic unit of local government, that is, a city or town (in Japanese, shi or machi).

However, during the discussion process, some proposed that central government rather than these local governments be the insurer, claiming that small municipalities would soon face financial problems.

Though it considered this proposal very carefully, the government concluded that municipalities were the best choice as new insurer, taking into account that they had traditionally and successfully operated most welfare services and they were familiar with the overall welfare system in which the new insurance scheme was to be established.

Coverage

The new insurance scheme covers only older people. Some expressed concern at coverage being limited in this way and argued that the new scheme should also cover people with disabilities. The government's position was that the scheme should exclusively cover older people on the grounds that, on one hand, a variety of public services are already provided for people with disabilities and, on the other hand, arriving at a definition of disability in the context of the new insurance scheme might prove too complicated.

Benefits

The long-term care insurance scheme is unique in that it will directly provide long-term care services for older people in need, rather than cash for the purchase of these or other services. However, there were those, particularly in rural areas, who insisted that some cash benefits be provided to persons engaged in long-term care of parents or parents-in-law; such benefits remain popular among caregivers.

On the other hand, women in urban areas generally disagreed with this opinion, asserting that cash benefits could in effect force women to stay at home to care for elderly family members. In addition, those in this group pointed out the possibility that cash benefits might not be used for their intended purpose. In the end, cash benefits were not included in the bill.

Outline of the New Insurance Scheme

The details of the new insurance scheme are described in the Long-Term Care Insurance Law and related regulations, to be effective in 2000. The outline of the new insurance scheme is as follows.

Insurer

Japan has a two-tier system of local government. One tier consists of 47 prefectures (in Japanese, ken) and the other is made up of some 3,200 municipalities: cities, towns or villages (shi, machi or mura). A municipality is the most basic unit of local government, responsible for various community services, including the operation of personal social services and the national health insurance scheme for unemployed and self-employed people.

In the year 2000, the municipalities will have authority and responsibility for the management and finance of the long-term care insurance scheme as a whole. They will provide insured persons with certain benefits and levy the necessary contributions.

Insured Persons

Under the Long-Term Care Insurance Law, there are two insured groups. The first comprises those aged 65 and over (the number in this category will be about 22 million in 2000) and the second those between the ages of 40 and 64. The former group are compulsory participants in the long-term care insurance scheme and are obliged to pay the contribution prescribed. The latter group are also compulsory participants but pay their contribution in addition to their regular contribution to the health insurance scheme to which they belong. Benefits for them are somewhat limited.

Benefits

The insured persons are entitled to various benefits from the new insurance scheme, paying as a rule only a 10 percent share of the costs. Benefits for persons aged 65 and over include:

1. welfare services for insured persons at home, such as home help, short-stay service and day service;

2. facility services at special nursing homes;

3. certain medical services at health service facilities and in sanatorium-type wards,1 and

4. daycare and home-visit nursing care for insured persons at home.

Benefits for insured persons between the ages of 40 and 64 are provided only in the case of particular diseases caused by ageing.

Cash benefits will not be provided to any family member engaged in caring for older people.

All medical services at health service facilities and at sanatorium-type wards which are financed by the Health and Medical Service Law for the Elderly, except for medical services at hospitals, are to be provided by the new insurance scheme.[2]

Examination of Need and Care Plan by Care Manager

Older people requiring any of the services provided by the insurance scheme must apply to the examination committee established by the insurer. The examination committee comprises professionals specializing in elder care.

The committee has the authority to decide, with the aid of a computerized evaluation program, how much long-term care is needed.

Applicants are to be grouped into six categories according to the extent of their need. If need is recognized by the committee, they will be informed of the cash value of the benefits available to them over a set period according to their category.

Once the application is approved, beneficiaries have a free choice of care manager, whom they ask to prepare on their behalf a care plan up to the approved benefit value. The care manager then makes the necessary arrangements for services according to the plan.

Since care managers are expected to play such an important role, they are required to pass a special qualifying examination.

Provision of Services

Service providers wishing to be engaged under the terms of the new insurance scheme must meet the requirement concerning necessary personnel and facilities and must be specified as an "appointed provider" by the prefectural government.

It has long been taken for granted that welfare services should be provided by governmental, quasi-governmental or non-profit organizations. On this basis, the government has been making every effort to develop the necessary service systems nationwide. Particularly over the past ten years, in accordance with the so-called Gold Plan (see Appendix), an extensive budget has been allocated to the field of welfare services for older people. In that time, welfare services for older people have rapidly developed to meet demand.

Future development

The government is now facing the need to reorganize the social security system because of its gigantic financial deficit. In this context, the health insurance system has also been reviewed and, at the same time, as mentioned above, reform of the Health and Medical Service Law for the Aged has been under discussion in the advisory council concerned.

One of the reasons for the introduction of the long-term care insurance scheme is to control the medical costs of older people by transferring as many inpatients as possible from hospital to home. From this point of view, some people insist on the need to amalgamate health insurance with long-term care insurance in the future. Other amendments rejected during the process of drawing up the bill are also likely to be tabled again for further discussion. The government recognizes the possibility of future amendments to the scheme, but also stresses the importance of launching the new scheme as smoothly as possible and on schedule.

However, most people interested in the new long-term care insurance program doubt whether traditional means will be enough to

Figure 8.3
Facility Services

(1) Special nursing homes for older people

Total accommodation
available in all welfare
facilities to older people
needing constant care
and for whom living at
home poses difficulties
(number of beds)

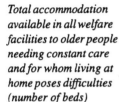
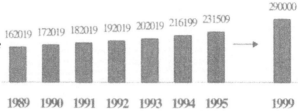

(2) Health service facilities for older people

Total accommoda-
tion available in all
facilities to older
people not needing
hospitalization but in
need of functional
training, nursing and
rehabilitation
(number of beds)

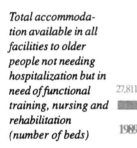
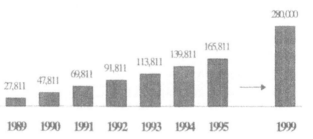

meet the vast demand which is likely to be set off by the implementation of the new scheme. They advocate full utilization of the so-called market mechanism. From this point of view, private enterprises will be recognized as appointed providers of some services—such as home help—as insurance benefits.

At the same time, it is suspected that excessive privatization of welfare services could lead to instability in the supply of necessary provision. This is particularly so in the area of facility services, where the sudden cessation of care for purposes linked to profitability might well affect the lives of those being cared for within the facility. Private enterprises are therefore not being authorized to play any part in the field of facility services for the time being.

The government remains subject to constant pressure from business circles demanding a more open market policy even in welfare services.

Coordination of Services between Regions by Implementation and Supporting Program

Each municipality responsible for running the new insurance scheme has to draw up an Implementation Program for the Long-Term Care Insurance Scheme, setting out the amount of services for older people it considers necessary within its boundaries.

However, it is feasible that a municipality could find itself unable to secure the requisite provision of services corresponding to its administrative area. For this reason, each prefectural government is expected to draw up a Supporting Program for the Long-Term Care Insurance Scheme, encompassing the municipalities it covers, in order to redress any imbalance of service provision between municipalities.

The prefectural government may reject an application for appointed provider status if the current provision of facilities is already at a satisfactory level.

Cost Calculation and Cost Sharing

Expenditure on services, except the portion borne by the insured person, is to be reimbursed to the service provider by the insurer. Expenditure is calculated on the basis of criteria set by the government.

The costs of services will be financed by copayments, insured persons' insurance contributions, and central or local government grants. Insured persons will pay 10 percent of the costs, though a copayment exceeding a certain amount will be refunded. The insurance scheme will bear the remaining costs. Half of the costs borne by the insurance scheme will be financed through contributions by the insured person and the other half through government grants.

One-third of contributions will be raised from insured persons aged 65 and over and the other two-thirds through the additional health insurance contributions of those aged between 40 and 64, at least for the time being. This ratio is subject to change on the occasion of a periodical financial review in accordance with the evolution of population ageing.

Approximate cost sharing:

Copayment by the insured individual: 10 percent

Contribution by insured persons aged 65 and over: 30 percent

Contribution by insured persons aged 40-64: 15 percent

Central government grant: 22.5 percent

Local government grant: 22.5 percent

Total cost: 100 percent

It was estimated that the total cost of the services provided through the new insurance scheme would come to over 4,000 billion yen at 1995 prices, but the cost is now being reviewed.

Review in Five Years

The introduction of the new long-term care insurance scheme means radical change in the current welfare system, and unpredictable problems will inevitably arise after its implementation. For this reason, the law prescribes a review and any necessary amendments to the scheme within five years after it comes into force.

Figure 8.4
Total Project Expenditure and National Expenditure on the New Gold Plan

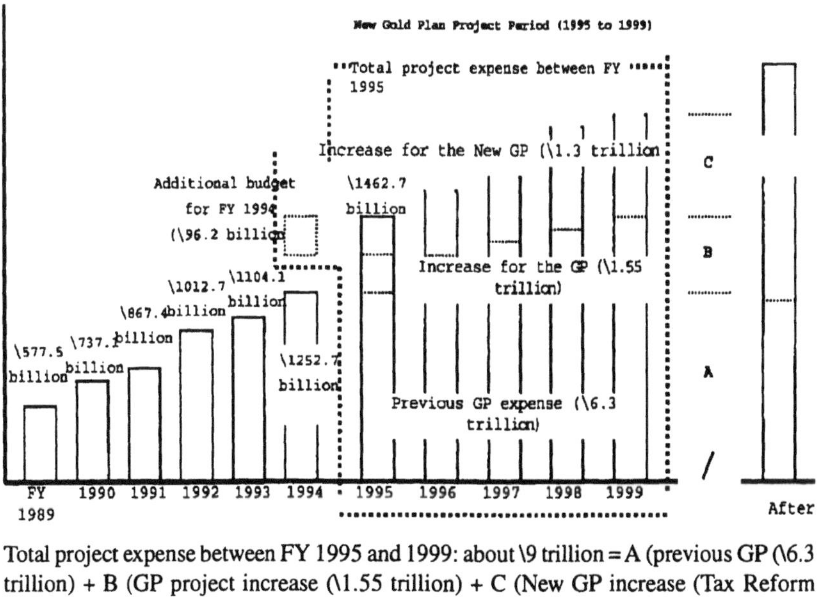

Total project expense between FY 1995 and 1999: about \9 trillion = A (previous GP (\6.3 trillion) + B (GP project increase (\1.55 trillion) + C (New GP increase (Tax Reform Frame\1.2 trillion + Additional budget for FY 1994 \0.1 trillion)
* To be considered during the deliberations on securing the necessary social security budget in connection with revisions to the consumption tax rate.

Figure 8.5
Target Areas Requiring the Urgent Development of Infrastructure for Care Services for Older People

(1) Home Help

Total staff who visit families with difficulties in providing care and household services for elderly relatives on a daily bases (number of helpers).

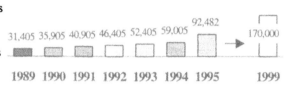

(2) Short Stay

Total accommodation within institutions such as special nursing homes which take care of older persons for a short time (number of beds).

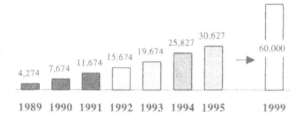

(3) Day Services/Daycare

Total number of facilities providing day services which are designed to provide the older persons with shuttle bus services or home-visit services to assist in bathing, meals, health check and training for daily activities. Daycare provides rehabilitation programs for older persons with dementia and having difficulties with daily activities due to strokes, etc. to maintain or recover their physcal function. (number of facilities).

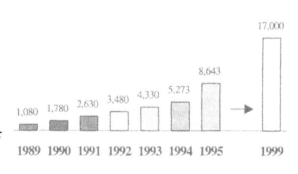

(4) In-home Care Support Centres

Total number of facilities providing easy access to expert counselling, guidance and ncessary health care services without need to go to the municipal office (number of stations).

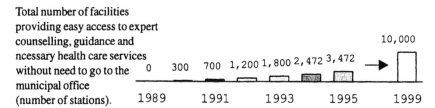

(5) Home-Visit Nursing Care Stations for Older People

Total number of stations which dispatch staff such as nurses to visit older people who are bedridden, etc., at home and provide various services focusing on nursing care (number of stations).

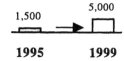

Appendix

Gold Plan (1989)

The Ten-Year Strategy to Promote Health Care and Welfare for the Elderly (the Gold Plan) was formulated in December 1989 with the agreement of three ministers: the Minister for Finance, Minister for Health and Welfare, and Minister for Home Affairs. This Gold Plan is an unprecedented gigantic ten-year project in the field of health and welfare for older people in Japan, with the total cost of six trillion (6,000,000,000,000) yen. The Plan originated from the objectives of the consumption tax which was introduced in April 1989. It consists of seven major projects such as urgent project to develop in-home welfare measures for older people on local government level, promotion of Campaign to Reduce the Number of Bedridden Elderly People to Zero, and urgent provision of service facilities, and sets numerical goals to be achieved by the fiscal 1999.

Practically, the Plan's goals as to in-home welfare are 100,000 home helpers, 10,000 day centers and 50,000 short-stay beds. As for facility measures, the goals are 240,000 beds at special nursing homes for the elderly, 280,000 beds at health service facilities for the elderly. In addition to the existing services facilities, the Plan welcomes new measures such as development of in-home care supporting centers, care houses and multipurpose senior centers. The Plan also aims to establish a functional training system as part of the "Campaign to Reduce the Number of Bedridden Elderly People to Zero, and a Cerebral Apoplexy Information System, to secure care-providing personnel resources and to enhance preventive education against cerebral apoplexy.

New Gold Plan (1994)

The result of a survey on local health and welfare plan for the older people, which was conducted in fiscal 1993, unveiled the fact that the Gold Plan should set higher goals than the original plan. For example, 68,000 more home helpers will be necessary and raising original numerical goals is also necessary for day services, short stays and special nursing homes for the older people. In order to revise the original plan as well as to reinforce the long-term care measures for the older people, the plan was revamped to the New Gold Plan in December 1994, based on the agreement of the three ministers involved with original Plan.

The New Gold Plan sets higher goals regarding infrastructure for long-term care services for the elderly, which was the priority project. It also indicates fundamental framework for future measures. Specifically, the basic concept for long-term care measures for older people are; (a) user-oriented services and support of self-sufficiency, (b) universalism, (c) provision of comprehensive services, and (d) community-oriented (regionalism). In addition, the new plan sets goals in the implementation of various measures such as reinforcement of community long-term care services for older people, enhancement of support measures for self-sufficiency as a follow-up on the "New Campaign to Reduce the Number of Bedridden Elderly People to Zero, measures for the senile elderly and development of service personnel resources as well as training. Aiming at efficient long-term care services available to any older people, the plan promotes comprehensive long-term care measures for older people including the establishment of a brand-new public long-term care system.

The total project cost for the New Gold Plan (fiscal 1995-1999) together with the Gold Plan, as a result, expanded to over nine trillion (9,000,000,000,000) yen.

Notes

1.   Sanatorium-type wards are medical care facilities for patients requiring long-term care, and are part of the institutional service in the long-term care insurance system.
2.   It is estimated that approximately 20 percent of all medical expenditure for older people will shift to the new scheme.

Part 5

New Institutional and Administrative Frameworks

9

Should Health Care be Part of the Social Security System or a Separate Scheme?

A. Ron

The interest today in the question of whether health insurance scheme should be part of a broad social security system or a separate institution is generated primarily by the nature of initiatives to establish new social health insurance schemes. The issue is particularly relevant in developing countries, which are only now starting social health insurance as the favored option to finance health care, with universal insurance coverage as the goal.

The optimal link between health care and the other social security branches will be considered later. Before doing so, it is important to look at the historic development of the linkage and the new initiatives. The early development of social security began with health care (Ron et al., 1990), as members of mainly occupational guilds created mutual societies to use pooled funds in times of distress due to sickness. Again stemming from a labor-related development, work injury programs were established to assure employer liability for medical services for work related injuries and illness (Social Security Programmes throughout the World, 1995). Over time, there was recognition of the rationale for using the social security framework to provide income replacement throughout other contingencies associated with the loss of earning capacity, including old age, invalidity and maternity. It was natural that all these social security branches, which by nature required the similar functions of registration and regular payment of contributions, usually shared between employers and workers, would be combined under a single administration.

In this development, it has always been clear that management of the health care component had special needs and warrants a separate administration within the broad social security scheme. As opposed to other social security branches, the broad categories of benefits may be defined within different classifications, such as ambulatory and hospital-based care, or preventive, curative and rehabilitative care, or as primary, secondary and tertiary care. Whatever spectrum or classification is applied, the specific services covered are constantly changing. Adaptations are necessary to deal with recognized developments of modern medical and health technology, as well as changes in the demography and disease patterns of the insured populations.

The predictability of the volume of specific or the constantly adaptation of the range of benefits is certainly not the same as for pensions, nor any other social security benefit. It has always been recognized that health insurance requires more complicated actuarial analyses, taking into account utilization and health care cost trends which are not limited to predictions of long-term demographic changes. As a result of recognition of these characteristics, the health care administration in social security systems generally had a separate organizational component, staffed by medical professionals.

Within the merged systems, the accounting functions for each of the benefits was generally kept separate. That is, contributions to health care or to pension funds were maintained within funds earmarked for each purpose, according to the specific contribution revenues and the expenditures for the specific benefits. There are indeed frequent misconceptions on this aspect, where it is erroneously assumed that merged social security systems mean merged funds.

While most early initiatives for social insurance development in all the benefit branches were linked to labor development, these did not come at a time when the majority of workers were salaried or when distinctions were made between formal and informal labor sectors. This point should be stressed, as it could lead to another erroneous assumption, which is that merged social security systems are predominantly found in countries in which most of the population fit in categories of active and retired formal sector workers and their dependents.

Table 9.1 shows the institutional and administrative structure of social health insurance in a number of countries, as last reported (Social Security Programmes throughout the World, 1997). The countries, listed alphabetically, were included if social health insurance has been formally established through national decree or legislation. The limited number of countries spans early and later development in different parts of the world.

It is indeed difficult to find any pattern in the current institutional arrangements. Social health insurance systems operating as part of broad social security systems, under the supervision of the Ministry of Labour and Social Security, may have health care functions, including the direct provision of health care in hospitals and clinics owned by the scheme, as in Turkey. Social health insurance in Greece is organized within the broad social security system, but under the supervision of the Ministry of Health, Welfare and Social Security. Chile on the other hand, has separate systems for health and the other social security branches. Health care is further divided into two systems, and following amendments in recent years, individuals can choose to enroll in either system. The public system, under the National Health Service, covers public and private sector workers, and persons receiving other social security benefits, such as pensions, work injury, unemployment or family allowance benefits. The private system covers active workers and their dependents.

It may therefore not be useful to look for patterns in current institutional arrangements and then attempt to determine optimal models for the institutional structure of social health insurance. Understanding the etiology of the schemes and the social, economic and political trends in the specific country, as well the source of new initiatives to develop health insurance, may be far more important.

The initiatives for new social insurance schemes are occurring in countries in which the majority of workers are not salaried, and are in what we term the informal sector. Such initiatives are also developing in countries going through the transition from centrally planned to market economies, where several other factors come into play. Economic development policies may seek to shift the burden for workers' welfare from the enterprise level to broader pooling potential (Hu, 1998; Hu, 1999). The introduction of social health insurance constitutes both a pooling mechanism and a new type of partnership between employer and workers in sharing contributions,

Table 9.1

Institutional Arrangements of Social Health Insurance in Selected Countries

Country	Social Security System	Health Care System	Comments
Argentina	National Social Security Administration: general supervision and administration	Ministry of Health and Social Action: general supervision National Institute of Social Services: co-ordination and administration	Minister of Labour and Social Security: maternity benefits
Australia	Department of Social Security: administration		Health Insurance Commission: administration of medical and health benefits
Belgium	Ministry of Social Affairs, Public Health, and the Environment: general supervision		National Sickness and Invalidity Insurance Institute: co-ordination for cash and medical benefits
Brazil	Ministry of Social Security and Social Assistance: general supervision National Social Security Institute: administration of benefits	Ministry of Health: general supervision Unified system for the administration of cash benefits for health	
Chile	Ministry of Labour and Social Welfare through Superintendent of Social Security: general supervision of old system Superintendent of Social Security:: general supervision of new system	Ministry of Health: general supervision of public system National Health Services: administration of benefits and services Superintendent of Health Institutions: oversees private system	
Costa Rica	Costa Rican Social Insurance Fund: administration		Fund owns and operates hospitals and clinics
Finland	Ministry of Social Affairs and Health: general supervision of private sector social security pension programme, sickness and maternity programme Social Insurance Institution: administration of pension and sickness programme		
Greece	Ministry of Health, Welfare, and Social Security: general supervision Social Insurance Institute: administration of programme of workers' pension and medical benefits		Institution operates hospitals and clinics.
Slovenia	Institute for Pension and Disability Insurance : general supervision	National Institute of Medical Insurance: sickness	Ministry of Labour, Family and Social Affairs: maternity
Turkey	Ministry of Labour and Social Security: general supervision Social Insurance Institution: administration		Institution operates hospitals.

usually in a progressive manner. A health insurance fund with defined revenues also requires the definition of specific benefits, with equity as a stated objective. The system therefore relieves both employer and worker from the personal component in covering costs on an episodic basis. As long as the worker is entitled to benefits, their cost is not dependent on the financial state of the enterprise at the time of use of care or payment. From the health system viewpoint, the regular contributions create a fund, which facilitates the prediction of revenues for health care providers, and therefore have the potential for better planning of services. To some extent, some governments therefore see the development of health insurance as a catalyst to change in the transition period (Ensor, 1998).

At the same time, the transition may have other implications, which affect the implementation of the new social insurance schemes. The target population in transition economies includes many household heads who may be in the process of losing both job security and some social protection as they shift from salaried state employment to a far less controlled and less protective private sector. In those countries, past practices may in fact contribute to better understanding of the value of social protection mechanisms, for both short-term benefits such as health care and long-term income replacement in old age. However, this former public sector population may be far less familiar with regular contributory mechanisms, which include deductions from their monthly salaries or earnings. They may also have a general tendency to stay clear of new measures which require initial registration, based on a perception that these will be linked to the other tax collection systems, such as taxes on their new incomes.

The recent initiatives to introduce health insurance are for the most part coming from government ministries responsible for health care. These countries generally have public health care delivery systems, owned and operated by government at national, regional and local levels. Faced with pressures to reduce public spending, the governments are seeking options to shift from the responsibility to directly finance health care, to the establishment of alternative financing mechanisms (Ron, 1998). In the process of determining the mechanisms, some form of cost-sharing by the consumers or the general population is usually an integral feature. These same ministries are also looking for alternative and additional sources of funding for their health care facilities, as these countries are generally characterized by government provision of both public and personal health care services.

Social health insurance may have been considered as the optimal mechanism right from the start of a health care financing reform process. It is more likely that health insurance is given serious and then very urgent attention when it is clear that other cost-recovery methods, such as user fees for health care at the time of use, either give very low yield or are politically unpopular and expensive to control.

All this means that pressures to introduce health insurance are now coming mainly from government ministries of health and not from labor organizations. In some countries, the pressures are part of overall health care reform conditions advised by international lending agencies. In such situations, there may be some lack of understanding of the principles of social health insurance and social security in general, so that the development of health insurance is considering simply a financing mechanism rather than a form of social protection.

There may be parallel interest in such social protection from previously excluded population groups in countries in which existing social security schemes may not have been able or willing to cope with extension of coverage to new populations. However, these tend to be isolated initiatives from communities, cooperatives or nongovernment organizations, as described in the chapter on the extension of health insurance coverage in the informal sector.

To deal with the question of whether social health insurance should be part of social security systems or not, we should review the issues in terms of political ideology, compliance and administrative efficiency.

Political Ideology

Within the context of political ideology, we should first consider the relationship between social health insurance and other social security benefits for the target population. If we take the broader approach to social safety nets, health insurance is one part of a spectrum of social protection measures. If it is put in place on its own to assure (financial) access to health care for the working population, including dependent children, we will need to look at what income-replacement or other social safety nets will cover the non-economically active populations. These include retired workers, invalids or unemployed for various reasons as well as the very low-income population. Access to health care has its obvious merits, both in terms of providing protection and as a mechanism for stable health care financing. However, its introduction should not ignore the need to assure income during the same contingencies of old-age, disability, maternity and unemployment.

The worst scenario, as has occurred in several countries, is competition between different government ministries, to push for the passage of legislation for their specific social security branch first, without attempting a coordinated approach. The competition is not necessarily related to the administrative capacity to manage any particular benefit branch, or from real needs of the population. It basically stems from the knowledge that contributions mean increased labor costs and deductions from salaries, both of which are limited in scope and essentially unpopular.

In the first chapter of this book, dealing with the extension of social health insurance coverage, the relative attractiveness of health care over the obviously less frequently needed, or long-term, social security benefits was discussed. Even with limited understanding of what social security benefits people are more interested in at different stages of the lifespan, we need to be careful about the decision to establish and operate separate schemes for the different social security branches. The real question is what will a separate system mean for social safety nets in the long run? A pragmatic question is whether a separate health care scheme will also manage the short-term cash income replacement during illness? The more important issue, however, is whether the scheme will defer the introduction of long-term social security benefits, mainly in the form of income replacement.

Compliance

Another pragmatic issue is compliance in registration and contribution collection if the social health insurance is a separate institution. Compliance probably depends more on internal pressures of the insured to be entitled to specific benefits than on external pressures through inspection and sanctions. If a pension system is well established, workers may be far more interested in the contribution base and consequent deduction for their contributions, as this will have direct bearing on how much they receive as income on retirement. The monthly pensions are usually a percentage of reported salary, adjusted for the number of years of work, and retired workers would then receive a pension directly linked to their own salaries. Health insurance contributions may be progressive, that is, the insured will pay according to means, but the use of benefits should be according to need. That is, the workers, both active and retired and their dependents will be entitled to the same benefits, regardless of their past incomes.

This fact in itself may work to the disadvantage of compliance in the deductions of contributions that are only for health insurance. The worker will obviously prefer to have a lower amount deducted if the amount of contribution does not endanger the potential receipt of benefits. Therefore, the same mechanism for deduction of contributions from the same salary base will be a factor in favor of combining health insurance with other social security branches.

The same kind of approach can be applied when looking at limitations on entitlement. For health insurance, the member is generally covered for three to six months after the last contribution has been paid. If this period is longer, the qualifying terms or limitations of new membership may be applied. The need for health insurance benefits is not predictable in most cases, just as the nature and volume of health care that may be required for any episode or illness is not generally known before the health care is actually sought. In theory, the insured persons, and those on whose behalf payments are made, are therefore concerned that payments should be kept up regularly and not fall behind or be neglected for long periods. This is quite different for pensions, beginning with the fact that retirement is generally planned. The entitlement to pension or provident fund benefits is usually 120 months or ten years of contributions to the fund. It is not unusual to find that insured persons who have exceeded this essential contribution period will favor discontinuing their payment until they can claim the retirement benefit, thereby weakening the actual fund. This is an increasingly common form of non-compliance, and it comes at a time when retirees may expect to live longer than the previous generation.

The effect of this non-compliance is even greater if we consider that salaries and incomes, and subsequently contributions, are likely to be higher in the more senior years of employment. If indeed, the social security mechanism has been put in place to have the means to provide income replacement in old age over an increasing number of years, any such discontinuation should be avoided. Stable income in old age is an obvious way to reduce the effects of deterioration in health associated with poverty in old age. Again, this factor strengthens the argument for a single registration and contribution collection mechanism.

Administrative Efficiency

The obvious advantage of having health insurance within the broad social security system is the registration of the insured and the continued collection of contributions. As long as employers are partners in the payment of contributions, they will be reluctant to have duplicate requirements for registration of their workers, and the regular deductions and remittance of contributions. Combined management of these functions should provide administrative efficiency regardless of the advantages above related to compliance. At a time when even well-established schemes face deficits and look for savings, it seems all the more important to combine at least these administrative functions. The administrative efficiency and opportunities for effective monitoring and cost control also relate to high cost information systems, particularly those dealing with membership database management and the recording of the use of benefits.

In Japan, an employer or group of employers are permitted to establish a health insurance society, which operates as a health insurance plan contracted out of the state health care plan. The extent of risk pooling is obviously limited in such societies, and the relatively small number of insured persons may hamper favorable conditions in relationships with health care providers. Contribution income has been decreasing because of the state of the economy, while the costs of the health care benefits continue to increase. In 1998 (IBIS Briefing Service, April, 199, page 22), about 55 percent of the 1.813 health insurance societies had a deficit. In response to the situation, from March 1999, the Ministry of Health and Welfare allowed employers to terminate their health plans and register their workers in the state system. Undoubtedly, administrative efficiency has played a part in determining the merits ᵢf the change in regulations.

The policy on health insurance development should also deal with whether it is intended from the beginning to have a single national scheme or whether a pluralistic approach will be taken, in which case there may be multiple schemes, linked to specific communities, occupational sectors or other forms of association. If the approach is pluralistic, there may be a need for a stronger health insurance policy unit in the Ministry of Health, with a national umbrella agency to coordinate and support development of the various schemes. Such an agency can indeed provide support through the sharing of administrative functions, including provider contractual arrangements, and share development experiences. If the social health insurance scheme is developed as a separate institution, the next question relates to where it should it be (a) directly in the Ministry of Health, (b) a separate agency supervised by the Ministry of Health, or (c) completely independent of any government ministry. The decision of where to locate health insurance may involve another set of issues, which are in fact some of the neglected areas in the health system reform process.

The situation in most countries with acute health care financing problems is that the Ministry of Health is still the main provider of health services, including public preventive services and personal curative care. One possibility is that the Ministry of Health recognizes the potential for additional funding for health, but then sees these revenues within the narrow concept of funds to replace the depletion in the health care budget for its own hospitals. That in itself may be the reality, and indeed one of the objectives of health insurance. However, such a limited focus can lead to a negative process in which government providers work to generate income through the provision of unnecessary health services, at the expense of the government health insurance fund. The situation is aggravated when these hospitals are required to continue providing care "free of charge" to civil servants, without the necessary transfers from other government agencies, for example, the Ministry of Education which employs teachers. A new health insurance mechanism for private sector workers is often first perceived by both public and private providers as a generous third-party payor with very little control over its expenditures. The utilization and cost control mechanisms required to monitor and prevent this situation are usually beyond the capacity of all the partners. Obviously, appropriate provider payments systems and contractual agreements between the fund and providers can go a long way to prevent this situation, and this area is dealt with elsewhere in this publication.

In this context, we may also find ethical concerns regarding the use of funds accrued through regular prepayment of contributions by the insured, or members of the health insurance scheme. The same concern applies regardless of whether the scheme is financed by contributions paid by employers and employees, or only by individuals or households. If the issue were put to the ethical test, the prevailing argument would be that such contributions should certainly be pooled to enable the greatest possible sharing of risks and funds, but should not be used for those who do not contribute at all. Indeed, the services provided by health insurance schemes, which have set up direct delivery systems, are usually jealously guarded by the members, who are reluctant to open the doors of these facilities to non-insured populations.

If the initiative to introduce health insurance comes from the Ministry of Health, it may be assumed that it should be part of the Ministry of Health. While there may be advantages in terms of familiarization with the specific nature of health care benefits, there are reasons why it may not be advisable to develop social health insurance as a unit within a Ministry of Health. In many countries, administrative capacity in health ministries is not strong, and is further hampered by the operation of a wide range of under-funded facilities to provide health care. The statutorial functions of health ministries are often compromised because of this administrative load. A significant part of the statutory functions includes accreditation and regulation of health care professionals and facilities. If the health insurance system is set up within the Ministry of Health, there may be serious delays in determining both the standards and the process for accreditation. The major reason is that many government facilities, built decades ago but now suffering from years of weak maintenance, do not meet the requirements for accreditation, as developed in the context of up-to-date criteria. If the health insurance system is outside the Ministry of Health, there could at least be more pressure to have criteria in place and to improve government facilities as an integral part of the implementation of the system.

Ministries of Health have a wide range of administrative functions, many of which are not specific to the health or medical field. They often employ large numbers of health workers, and may in fact constitute one of the largest employers in the country. However, they tend to have less contact and experience in the registration of enterprises or employers, and the routine collection of contributions outside their own government institutions. The section above on compliance detailed the complexities of these functions and the potential negative impact of weakness in these functions on the viability of a health insurance scheme.

Regardless of the level of contributions to a social health insurance scheme, the revenue from these contributions constitutes a regular and usually predictable source of income into a separate account. The fund established generally has allocations for administration, information systems and communications. The same budgetary allocation features often do not apply in a government ministry, particularly in an era of pressure to reduce public spending and when administrative functions are chronically under-funded. Such differences in the budgetary environment can lead to negative relationships between the various operational units in the Ministry of Health, to the extent that growth of the health insurance scheme is hampered rather than promoted. When coordination is positive and growth of the social insurance is a common goal, it becomes difficult to separate the functions of monitoring and formulation of health insurance policy from the daily operation of the scheme. There may be fewer problems in social health insurance systems established under the supervision of the Ministry of Health but allowed to operate in an environment outside the physical structure of the ministry.

From the above, it appears that much of the debate on whether a separate health insurance system should be in or outside the Ministry of Health depends on the involvement of this in the provision of health care. The problems indeed seem to increase when the Ministry of Health, through national, provincial and local levels, is the sole or major provider of care. The health care reform process and the development of health insurance need to contend with the realistic future roles of the Ministry of Health. A basic question is whether a Ministry of Health should concentrate on the statutory and regulatory functions, with direct responsibility only for the provision of health services limited to public preventive services.

It is accepted that the Ministry of Health may indeed have to retain the function of direct provision of services for such populations, both public and personal in nature, until an adequate and balanced geographical distribution of resources is achieved. At this point, the use of the broad term "resources" should be noted, as it includes not only financial resources but also infrastructure and human resources for all population sectors. There may be some expectation in the Ministries of Health that direct ownership of operation of facilities can be shifted or taken over by private initiatives, and that the revenues accrued by health insurance schemes will cover the charges. However, it may take many years of carefully regulated development of private facilities and pricing policies before this can happen. In the interim stage, we are more likely to find that social health insurance based on affordable contributions for the majority of the population does not attract much private for-profit health care growth. Any planned hand-over of the delivery of care from government to non-government providers therefore needs to take this issue in consideration.

Conclusions

The more obvious advantages of having health insurance within the social security system are administrative efficiency and the potential to reach good compliance. A new social health insurance needs all the support and help it can get. This support will increase as the full range of objectives of introducing health insurance are realized, from the stable financing aspect to the potential for well-planned health system development. The final determinant, however, may be opportunistic and detached from broad social security principles. If the health insurance scheme is set up as a separate agency following genuine initiatives to solve the health care financing problem within a process of health care reform, this institution will still deserve all the support and collaboration it can get. Successful development of a separate institution, with credibility in the use of funds from a broad membership base, may be a significant contribution to reaching broader social safety goals.

The determination of whether a social health insurance scheme should be on its own or as part of a broad social security system is justifiably complicated. As seen above, the political ideology covers concerns for putting in place social protection in general, and not only the need or will to assure equity in access to health care through stable financing. The policy developed may include universal health insurance as the ultimate goal, and will deal with the partners in sharing the contribution burden. These may involve government, employers, and active and retired workers and their dependents at all income levels in the public and private sectors, as well as non-economically active individuals and disadvantaged populations. A rational decision on how to develop the scheme should come after clarification of who is paying, who is subsidizing whom, and the targets for the extent of the population to be covered over time.

References

Ensor, T., Thompson, R. 1998. "Health insurance as a catalyst to change in former communist countries?" *Health Policy*, 43: 203-218.

IBIS: International Benefits Information Service, April 1999 (page 22), USA, ISSN #0018-8611.

Hu, A., ILO, see Chapter 3 in this publication.

Hu, T.-W.; Ong, M., Lin, Z.-H., and Li, E. 1999. "The Effects of economic reform on health insurance and the financial burden for urban workers in China," *Health Economics* 8: 309-321

Ron, A., Abel-Smith, B., and Tamburi, G. 1990. *Health Insurance in Developing Countries: The Social Security Approach*, ILO Publication.

Social Security Programs Throughout the World—1995, Social Security Administration, Office of Research and Statistics, SSA Publication No. 13-11805, Research Report #64, July 1995, U.S. Government Printing Office, Washington, D.C.

Social Security Programs Throughout the World—1997, Social Security Administration, Office of Research and Statistics, SSA Publication No. 13-11805, Research Report #65, July 1997, U.S. Government Printing Office, Washington, D.C.

10

Private Participation in Supporting the Social Contact in Health: New Insights from Institutional Economics

A. S. Preker, A. Harding, and N. Girishankar

A Historical Snapshot

Since the beginning of written history, people have used home remedies, private healers, and the voluntary sector when they were ill.

Unlike this early private participation in health care, during the twentieth century, governments of most countries have become central to health policy, often engaging in both the financing and provision of a wide range of care. Today, most OECD countries have achieved universal access to health care through a mix of public and private financing arrangements and providers.[1]

Proponents of such involvement by the public sector in health care have argued their case on both philosophical and technical grounds. In most societies, care for the sick and disabled is considered an expression of humanitarian and philosophical aspirations. But one does not have to resort to moral principles or arguments about the welfare state to warrant collective intervention in health. The past 100 years is rich with examples of how the private sector and market forces alone fail to secure efficiency and equity in the health sector.

Largely inspired by Western welfare state experiences such as the British National Health Service and the problems of market failure, during the past 50 years, many low- and middle-income countries established state-funded health care systems with services produced by a vertically integrated public bureaucracy.

During the 1980s and 1990s, the pendulum began to swing back in the opposite direction. As in the case of the rise in state involvement in the health care, the recent cooling towards state involvement in health care and enthusiasm for private solutions has been motivated by both ideological and technical arguments.

During the Reagan and Thatcher Era,[2] the world witnessed a growing willingness to experiment with market approaches in the social sectors (health, education and social protection). This was true even in countries such as Great Britain, New Zealand and Australia that historically had been the bastions of the welfare state.

The political imperative that has accompanied liberalization in many former socialist states and the economic shocks in East Asia and Latin America have contributed to a global sense of urgency to reform inefficient and bloated bureaucracies and to establish smaller governments with greater accountability.[3]

In the health sector, all countries continue to face difficult challenges in meeting the health needs of their populations.[4] Despite a significant past engagement, it has become painfully clear that, although public sector involvement is essential for social protection, it is not enough by itself.[5] Governments everywhere are, therefore, reassessing when, where, how, and to what degree to intervene or to leave things to the private sector and market forces (see Figure 10.1).[6]

Figure 10.1
Government and Market Involvement in Health Systems

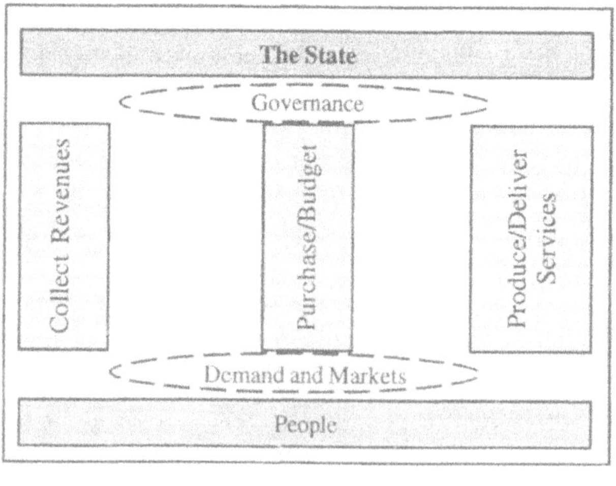

This chapter will demonstrate the need for a continued significant role of the state in the health sector.[7] But it challenges the principles and nature of public intervention pursued by many governments especially in the area of the public production of health services.[8] Using a framework based on recent developments in organizational economics, it argues a strong case for greater private participation in providing health services (rowing). At the same time, it advocates a more focused government engagement in securing equity, efficiency, and quality objectives through more effective policy making (steering), regulating, contracting, and ensuring that adequate financing arrangements are available for the whole population.

The Health Sector Dilemma

During recent years, there has been a surge in attempts to reform health care systems by exposing public services to competitive market forces, downsizing the public sector, and increasing private sector participation.[9] This trend is by no means only emblematic of the United States but reflects a worldwide approach to reforming public health care services.

Contrary to the assertions of some critics, in most cases these reforms are not intended to usurp the legitimate role of governments in the health sector. Economic theory provides ample justifications for such an engagement on both theoretical and practical grounds to secure:[10]

- efficiency since significant market failure exists in the health sector (information asymmetries; pubic goods; positive and negative externalities; distorting or monopolistic market power of many providers and producers; absence of functioning markets in some areas; and frequent occurrence of high transaction costs);[11] and

- equity since individuals and families often fail to protect themselves adequately against the risks of illness and disability on a voluntary basis due to shortsightedness (free-riding) and characteristic shortcomings of private health insurance (moral hazard and adverse selection).[12]

The range of possible actions that can be taken by governments to improve efficiency or equity—from least to most intrusive—is extensive. They include:[13]

- providing information to encourage behavior changes needed for improvements in health outcomes;

- developing and enforcing policies and regulations to influence public and private sector activities;

- issuing mandates or purchasing services from public and private providers; providing subsidies to directly or indirectly pay for services; and

- producing (in-house) preventive and curative services.

In many countries, for reasons of both ideological views and weak public capacity to deal with information asymmetry, contracting, and regulatory problems, governments often try to do too much—especially in terms of in-house service production—with too few resources and little capability.

Parallel to such public production, these governments often fail to:

- develop effective policies and make available information about personal hygiene, healthy life-styles, and appropriate use of health care;

- regulate and contract with available private sector providers;

- ensure that adequate financing arrangements are available for the whole population; and

- secure access to public goods with large externalities for the whole population.

Hence the dilemma that policymakers face throughout the world—although state involvement in the health sector is clearly needed, it is typically fraught with public sector production failure. The growing consensus is that to address this problem requires a better match between the role of state and the private sector, and their respective capabilities—getting the fundamentals rights. In most countries this means a re-balancing of what is already a complex mix of public and private roles in the health sector (see Figure 10.2).[14]

In the remainder of this section we will discuss the most significant sources of government production failure to which market-based solutions are being applied and the market imperfections that must be addressed to optimize complementarity between the two sectors.

The Nature of Government Failure

In recent years many attempts have been made to re-invigorate the public sector through "best practice" management techniques from the private sector and organizational reforms that attempt to replicate the incentive environment of the private sector.[15]

Figure 10.2
Range of Public and Private Configurations in the Health Sector

		Direct Fee	Risk-Pooling/Insurance Based		
		Out of Pocket	Private Insurance	Social Insurance	Social Insurance
Ownership of Health Services	Private				
	Mixed				
	Public				

These reforms have included efforts to strengthen the managerial expertise of health sector staff, both through training and recruitment policies. Frequently, attempts are also made to use business process re-engineering, patient-focused care, and quality improvement techniques. Such efforts have also included setting up clinical directorates, introducing improved information systems to facilitate effective decision-making, and performance bench marking.[16]

Why has the public sector been so resilient and unresponsive to these types of management and organizational reforms?[17] A review of theories regarding performance of governments of their multiple functions is needed to shed light on the profound nature of the structural problems involved. This review complements the well-developed theories of market failure provided by health economists.[18] In the following sections, we will explore the problems of poor public accountability, information asymmetry, abuse of monopoly power, failure to provide public goods, and a loss in strategic policy formulation that have parallels in market failure.

Problems Relating to Public Accountability

The first set of problems relates to the difficult task of translating preferences of individuals into public polity and getting that policy implemented. As we know, all public interventions involve transfers of benefits to some people and costs to others, that is, there are both winners and losers.[19]

Accountability means that government action accords with the will of the people it represents. Yet, since people's values are never perfectly homogeneous in any society, accountability will always be based on some imperfect rule about the aggregation of individual values or respect for minority interests.[20]

This raises several intractable procedural issues relating to accountability in the electoral process, taxation policies, contents of public spending programs, and vested bureaucratic interests.

Ballots are blunt instruments that cannot capture the full range of issues that may be bundled together at election time. The intensity of views on any one issue cannot be reflected. And, election promises are often not kept. So at best, public spending policies are a very imprecise reflection of social values.

Majority rule in itself can be a form of tyranny if applied strictly without constraints. Most democratic societies safeguard minority interests to some extent, but even with good intentions there are clearly both limits to practicality and desirability in this respect.

Finally, public servants may have strong conflicts between their assigned responsibilities to execute the collective will of the society they represent and their own interests. And, their political overseers may have strong vested interests that are different from those of the society that they represent.[21]

In an ideal setting, good public accountability would be secured through a large intersection (authorizing environment) between fairly homogeneous social values, a political agenda that reflects such values, and vested bureaucratic interests (see left box in Figure 10.3).[22] For example, there may be general social agreement on the need to protect the population against the financial consequences of illness through some sort of health insurance system. When the policies of the political party in power are consistent with such values and bureaucrats have the capacity to implement them the intersection will be large.

Figure 10.3
The Authorizing Environment Needed for Good Public Sector Accountability

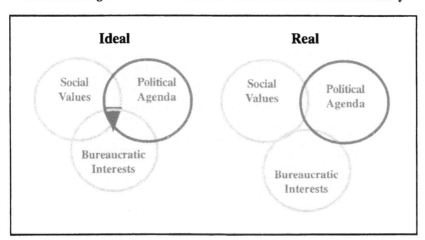

In the health sector, a further tension exists between the authorizing environment that is needed for good public accountability and the desire by most individuals for some sovereignty over their own health care. This leads to difficult dilemmas during the rationing of care or design of compulsory programs based on the application of some sort of majority rule that infringes on either perceived minority group rights or individual survival.[23] Normal rational individuals who may share social values about the need to ration health care resources often lose their commitment to such values when confronted by resource constraints in the face of serious illness or death.

Information Asymmetry in the Public Sector

Information asymmetry can occur in three major ways in the health sector—between the patient (public) and the health care professional; between the patient and the administrator or health care system; and between the health care professional and the administrator or health care system.

Patients know more about their symptoms than doctors but may—unwittingly or deliberately—not articulate this clearly. Doctors know more about the causes, prognosis, and effectiveness of available treatments but may not communicate this clearly to the patient. Or the patient may fail to understand the implications of what he/she is being told. For paternalistic reasons, the doctor may deliberately conceal information based on a judgment that the patient will not be able to cope with the full knowledge of his/or her ailment (e.g., a terminal cancer). Through self-selection, these problems are typically worse in the public sector that has to deal with large volumes of poorer and less educated patients.

When it comes to the interaction between the patient (public) and health care administrators, patients may try to avoid being excluded or paying higher health care premiums by choosing to conceal pre-existing conditions. Similarly, there is often a lack of information and understanding of available public programs. The benefit of gathering useful data about such programs is usually undervalued compared with its cost. Some of these programs may be too complex to fully understand even if information were available. Frequently there is a deliberated lack of transparency in the rationing of scarce resources.

Finally, some serious information asymmetries exist between health care providers and the administrators for which they work (or between the administrator and owner). The health care providers—as advocates for patients—have a much better understanding of legitimate needs or demand. The administrator has a much better understanding about the supply and cost of available resources, but knows little about the appropriateness of a selected intervention, or if it performed well. The well-know information advantage of the doctor to the patient is not solved by the existence of a public employer or administrator who knows even less about the interaction between the patient and the health care provider.

Associated Higher Transaction Costs

Such information asymmetries add to agency costs in terms of the structuring, monitoring, and bonding contracts among agents and principals with conflicting interests.[24] Private firms that are concerned with profits have a very strong incentive to limit the agency costs related to information asymmetry.[25] Public agencies that are not held to a clear "bottom line" due to unspecified social functions and many complex sources of subsidies do not receive clear signals about the agency cost of such information asymmetry.

Not surprisingly, many public health care facilities in low- and middle-income countries do not keep detailed patient records, do not know statistics, and do not know the unit costs of the procedures they are using or illnesses they treat. Hospitals are often not doing what policymakers or administrators would like, or what they think they should be doing. And, doctors working is such public hospitals maintain an information advantage that gives them a great deal of latitude to pursue their own interests. Paradoxically, since public systems often give less leverage to beneficiaries than private systems give clients, patients may be less able to use the information they do possess to influence their own treatment.

Potential for Corruption

What is worse than this ignorance by default due to information asymmetry, is the information problem that is actually deliberately engineered by politicians, bureaucrats, organizations, and health care providers that are entrusted with public accountability.

Although deliberate deception and fiscal fraud is usually sanctioned severely, it is much harder to hold the public sector accountable for petty abuses, avoidance, and obfuscation. Such deception may take the form of hidden costs, subsidies, cost shifting, or inflation. Or it may occur as an amplification of benefits, exaggeration of the consequences of alternatives, or claiming credit for activities that originate elsewhere.

Given the complex nature of health care it is not hard to imagine the considerable scope for patients and the public being misled or defrauded in the health sector.

The Abuses of Public Monopoly Power

Monopoly power occurs when the public sector gets involved in the production of health services for four reasons. This may be due to: (a) legal restrictions against competition; (b) access to subsidized capital and revenues creating an uneven "playing field"; (c) distribution of goods and services at below costs to achieve equity goals; or (d) production of public goods or goods where markets are not viable.

When—in addition to the above accountability, and information problems—the public sector enjoys monopoly power, those who work for it are given considerable scope for abusing this monopoly power through the extraction of rents, internal distribution of "slack to employees, and lowering of quality."

Public monopolies exhibit the usual negative features. First, monopoly suppliers often reduce output and quality, while raising prices. The excess in prices over and above what the market would normally bear—"rents"—leads to allocative inefficiency or a net dead-weight welfare loss to consumers who have to forgo the consumption of other goods.

A manifestation of such rents is the informal user charges that are commonly levied on patients and their families in publicly provided health facilities. In many countries, these rents are not limited to doctors accepting bribes or peddling influence (allowing privileged patients to circumvent the usual rules on resource allocation, to receive preferential treatment, and to cut waiting time). It also includes charges levied by other salaried workers for a wide variety of items such as toilet paper, and clean linen, or patients and their families having to buy food, drugs, and medical supplies.

In a recent study on corruption from around the world, such abuses in publicly run health services ranked as number one in terms of the burden that this places on households.[26] When they can afford it, patients often prefer to pay formal charges in the private sector to such rents in the public sector. Taxpayers being charged twice for low quality services and such abuses have little recourse other than the blunt and often ineffective instrument of voting power.

Second, monopoly suppliers have strong incentives to lower expenditures through decreased output when staff benefit from the financial residuals. Although public organizations cannot legally distribute such residuals outside the organization to shareholders, there are several ways that they can be internally consumed. First, executives often receive generous social benefits and travel (perks). Second, time-keeping is often not enforced rigorously (doctors often work short hours in public institutions). Third, some of the residual may be used to pursue personal agendas (discretionary spending on special projects and research).

Failure of Critical Policy Formulation

The most frequently cited reason for greater government involvement in the health sector is that when left to competitive forces and prices alone, in several other critical areas, the market does not lead to welfare enhancing production and allocation of a number of health care goods and services. These include:

- public goods (policy making and information)

- goods with large externalities (disease prevention)

- goods with intractable market failure (insurance)

It is therefore surprising that governments in the health sector often neglect the exact same three areas while they are busy with the production of curative services that the private sector could easily provide. More than half of the disease burden in Sub-Saharan Africa and South Asia could be addressed effectively through local adaptation of interventions such as immunization, integrated management of childhood illness, family planning, maternal and perinatal health care, food fortification, targeted nutrition programs, and school health. For example, infectious illnesses such as measles (which currently kills 1.1 million children a year) could also be eliminated or at least controlled at low levels with proper public policies.

The Theory of Market-Based Strategies

The current trend worldwide is to use three types of approaches to address the public sector failure problems described above in service delivery. They include increased:[27]

- exit possibilities (market consumer choice)

- voice (client participation)

- loyalty (hierarchical sense of responsibility)

These approaches are in descending order of strength. When possible you would always use exit (ceteris paribus), unless forced to use the weaker variants because the goods and services involved are not "marketable."

In this chapter we will focus mainly on the first of these options— the exit option. This approach relies on greater private sector participation, allowing clients and patients a choice or alternative to publicly provided services. Such exit options can be implemented in parallel with other public sector management reforms that increase voice and loyalty.

From Neoclassical Economics...

Critics of market-based approaches and advocates of strong public sector involvement often base their analysis on the shortcomings of markets health as outlined in neoclassical economics.[28]

One of the central tenets in favor of greater private sector participation is that in an optimally functioning market, competitive forces will lead to a more efficient allocation of resources—Pareto-optimal competitive equilibrium—than command economy or non-market solutions.[29] Under this neo-classical model—where there are a large number of firms and consumers and prices respond to the forces of supply and demand—a welfare-maximizing outcome can be predicted.[30]

Unfortunately the perfectly competitive Walrasian model relies on a number of assumptions that are often not present in real world situations, especially when applied to the health sector. These include:

- the goods involved behave like private goods (i.e., rivalness, excludability, and rejectability)

- rights can be perfectly delineated

- transaction costs are zero

In reality most health care activities do not involve goods that behave like perfect private goods. Many are not perfectly excludable but rather associated with complex externalities. Rights are often difficult to delineate, leaving residual claimants. And transaction costs are often high.

Therefore, although in a Pareto-optimal state, it would be impossible to make someone better off without making someone else worse off, it is hard to imagine a single public policy situation meeting this criteria.

The neoclassical paradigm clearly lays out the potential sources of market failure. The rationale for public ownership has been its effectiveness as a tool for pursuing social objectives in the presence of these market failures. This belief is based on a simple view of the relationship between ownership and control. Privately owned companies are generally believed to be profit-seeking—since by maximizing profits they maximize the benefits to their shareholders (or owners). In some cases, maximizing shareholder benefits is not seen to be maximizing the benefits to society as whole.

Broadly speaking, the two cases are: (a) circumstances where competitive solutions do not exist (natural monopoly); and (b) circumstances where they exist but are not efficient (because of externalities, nature of public goods, or significant information asymmetry). In health, this reasoning supports public intervention to address market failures with regard to both equity and efficiency.

Based on these insights, public ownership has been used as a tool to get the organization to replace the narrow interests of owners with the wider interests embodied in the state, to pursue social goals as opposed to private benefit (profit maximization).

...to the Economies of Organizations

Though neoclassical economics clearly lays out potential sources of market failure, the framework is actually silent on the critical issues of how to structure an effective institutional solution. The mechanism by which public ownership is supposed to lead to maximization of social goals is nowhere precisely defined. In fact, neoclassical economics is essentially "institution free."[31] Recently, this vacuum has been filled, with the development of analytical tools for understanding the effectiveness of different ownership and governance arrangements.

Much progress has been made in identifying the key factors causing wide variations in performance of organizations. The developments most relevant for understanding the advantages and disadvantages of different arrangements for service delivery come from principal-agent theory, transaction cost economics, property rights and public choice theory. These fields are often grouped together under the title "economics of organizations"—and all deal with considerations of information, motivation and innovation and the implications for how productive activity can best be organized.

The traditional rationale for public ownership was based on a simplistic model of individual behavior-presupposing that the objectives of the government and the objectives of the managers running public organizations were identical. Policymakers assumed that if managers were told to pursue the public interest, they would be able to determine what that meant and would have the necessary incentives to implement it.

In practice, the vagueness of the objectives and the difficulty of precisely determining and monitoring output has proved "inimical to the efficient management of the (sectors) concerned."32 Public ownership removed the opportunistic profit maximizer—but the civil servant or politician has turned out to be no "high custodian of public interest," instead, they have often tended to pursue their own private benefits. The economics of organization directly addresses the issue of how best to structure organizations that consist of individuals pursuing their own self interest.

Agency theory. This framework highlights the need to reconcile divergent interests among individuals under conditions of widespread uncertainty and uneven access to information. The key relationship is modelled as occurring between a principal and an agent. The principal needs the efforts and expertise of the agent but has only limited ability to monitor the agent's actions or evaluate whether the final outcome was satisfactory.

The agency literature surveys the range of contracts, such as payment and monitoring arrangements, observed in the economy as attempts to align incentives and reward cooperation between self-interested but interdependent individuals.[33] The need for incentive alignment is pervasive in the health sector: the relation between patient and physician is a classic case of the principal-agent structure. Physicians and hospital managers have divergent interests and different competencies, yet they need one another. Most important for our review is the principal-agent relation between the government owner and hospital management.

Governments, like firms, must design evaluation and reward mechanisms to obtain high quality performance regardless of whether they are contracting with outside providers/suppliers, or with employees. Several studies have generalized the agency insight from the employment context to the full range of relationships that make up the firm-now conceptualized as a nexus of many contracts.[34] This conceptualization has increased the understanding of ownership and governance by clarifying the relationship between suppliers of capital, both equity shareholders and bond debt holders, and the managers of the firm. By illuminating critical elements of relations between owners and firms, this analysis has also improved understanding of the governance relations between governments and public service providers.

The rise and dominance of the modern corporation is attributed to its successful governance structure. This structure allows professional managers to be assigned decision rights and performance incentives, though they bear relatively little financial risk. At the same time, risk is borne by diversified investors, who need not assume control.

From the perspective of agency theorists, the range of organizational arrangements is interpreted as the outcome of a competitive process in which particular forms survive where they best control the technological, informational, and motivational sources of agency failure. Much of the momentum behind reforms which create new service delivery arrangements is generated by this belief that contractual and governance arrangements developed under the competitive pressures of markets can usefully be applied to public sector organizations.

Another insight from the principal-agent framework relates to moral hazard. Moral hazard refers to the inefficient behavior under a contract, arising from the differing interests of the contracting parties, which persists only because one party to the contract cannot tell for sure whether the other is honoring the terms of the contract. For example, in most jobs it is impossible to measure accurately the marginal product of each worker. Employers might attempt to measure employees' output by relying on proxies of performance, such as reports of supervisors. However, this often generates goal-displacing behaviors. Employees focus inordinate effort on the elements of their work that are rigorously monitored and shirk where monitoring is less rigorous.

This structural problem is particularly prevalent in health, where many of the outputs or features that owners or buyers care most about are unobservable-making it extremely difficult to effectively focus on either hospital or employee activities.

Transactions cost economics. Transaction cost economics has contributed greatly to understanding alternative governance structures, particularly the differences between the nature of markets (inter-organizational relationships) and firms (intra-organizational relationships). This contrasts with the agency theory view of the firm as a nexus of contracts-which downplays the distinctive features of internal organization versus market exchange.

Transaction cost economics emphasizes the limitations of contracts and the need for more flexible means of coordinating activity-that is, internal organization. Because of the cognitive limits of economic agents, their willingness to pursue self-interest, and the unforeseeable changes in the environment, every contract, even the most detailed, is inherently incomplete. None can fully anticipate and accommodate the differing interests of the negotiating parties. Formal contracts need to be supported by organizational means of responding to unforeseen events and adjudicating the problems they create. Integrating activities inside a single organization can bring this about in many contexts.

This theory sheds most light on firm boundaries and the conditions under which it is best to arrange activities within a hierarchy versus interacting in a market with suppliers or other contractors. More generally, vertically integrated organizations, simple "spot" contracts, franchises, or joint ventures are interpreted as discrete structural alternatives-each offering different advantages and disadvantages for effective governance.[35]

Governance arrangements are evaluated by comparing the patterns of costs generated for planning, adapting and monitoring production and exchange.[36] Unlike public organizations, private firms have the flexibility (indeed the requirement) to adjust their governance structure to changes in the market environment-making them fruitful targets for identifying "better practices" for governance arrangements.

Vertically integrated (within firm) organization arises as a response to problems with market contracting. The firm substitutes low-powered incentives, like salaried employment, for the markets' high-powered incentives of profit and loss. Vertical integration permits the details of future relations between suppliers (including employees), producers, and distributors to remain unspecified; differences can be adjudicated as events unfold. Vertical integration (or unified ownership) pools the risks and rewards of various activities undertaken by the organization, and can facilitate the sharing of information, the pursuit of innovation, and a culture of cooperation.

Notwithstanding these positive features, vertical integration suffers from characteristic weaknesses as a mechanism of governance. The two most prominent are the weakening of incentives for productivity and the proliferation of influence activities (see Box 10.1). The weak incentives come from people capturing less and less of the gains of their own efforts as rewards and losses are spread throughout the organization. Despite its focus on the contracting problems that motivate internal organization, transactions cost economics views

---

Box 10.1
Influence Activities

An important issue related to moral hazard and the structure of organizations is influence activities and the associated costs, known as influence costs.[37] Recent analysis has shed much light on the propensity of publicly owned service delivery organizations to capture inordinate portions of the sector budget, as well as their ability to influence sector policy to their benefit - often at the expense of public interest.

In the health sector, provider organizations expend effort to affect decisions regarding the distribution of resources or other benefits among providers to their benefit. These "influence activities" occur in all organizations, but countervailing forces are particularly weak in public service delivery structures-and influence costs are one of the most important costs of centralized control. Evidence of such "influence activities" is seen in public utilities where monopolies are often maintained to protect low productivity of state-owned enterprises from competition from more efficient producers. In the health sector, the tendency to allocate resources to tertiary and curative care at the expense of primary, preventative and public health is evidence of similar "capture."

It is important to note that the costs of these activities include both the losses associated with the poor resource allocation decisions as well as the loss associated with the efforts exerted to capture the rents. These costs can be reduced when there is no decision maker with authority to make decisions that service providers can easily influence, and this condition can sometimes be brought about by creating legal or other boundaries between the policymaker, funder and the service provider unit. Many organizational reforms have attempted to diminish these activities. Examples include reforms separating the policy maker from the payer from the provider in public service delivery, as well as privatization of utilities.

---

vertical integration as the governance mechanism of last resort. Even in the many instances where policy objectives imply that spot market transactions aren't desirable, contractual networks, virtual integration, franchising, or concessioning will out-perform unified ownership arrangements.

Property rights theory. Property rights theory looks at the same incentive issues from a slightly different perspective. Since private ownership appears to have strong positive incentives for efficiency, property rights theorists have attempted to find out why (see Box 10.2). Explanations have focused on two issues: the possession of residual decision rights and the allocation of residual returns.[38]

Residual rights of control are the rights to make any decisions regarding an asset's use not explicitly contracted by law or assigned to another by contract. The owner of an asset usually holds these rights-though the owner or the law may allocate many rights to others.[39] The notion of ownership as residual control is relatively clear for a simple asset like a car. It gets much more complicated when applied to an organization such as a firm. Large organizations bundle together many assets, and who has which decision rights may be ambiguous. For example, do the directors of a firm have the right to accept a takeover offer without soliciting competing bids?

In addition to residual decision rights, an owner holds the rights to residual revenue flows from his assets. That is, the owner has the right to whatever revenue remains after all funds have been collected, and all debts, expenses, and other contractual obligations have been paid out. Just as the allocation of residual control can be fuzzy in the case of firms (because rights of control of different categories of decisions may be poorly specified or may lie with various parties), the notion of residual returns is fuzzy as well.

One problem is that recipients of residual returns may vary with the circumstances. When a firm is unable to pay its debt, increases in its earnings may have to be paid to the lenders. In those cases, the lenders are the residual claimants. Firms may pay bonuses, increase workers' pay, and promote more workers' into higher-ranking, higher paying jobs when performance is up. So, some of the workers share in the residual returns of the firm. It is the pairing of residual returns and residual control which is key to the incentive effects of ownership. These effects are very powerful because the decision-maker bears the full financial impact of his choices.

Political choice theory. Political choice theory has strongly influenced organizational reform. A central tenet of public choice is that all human behavior is dominated by self-interest. Individuals are viewed as rational utility maximizers. Public choice theorists apply this model to understanding how individuals will react in different institutional settings with different incentive structures. They also study collective action problems-that is, problems that arise when the pursuit of individual interests produces sub-optimal outcomes for the collectivity.

This field focuses on the self-interested behavior of politicians, interest groups, and bureaucrats, and studies the implications for effective government and the size of government. Bureaucrats, attempting to maximize their budgets, will acquire an increasing share of national income. As a result, the state will grow well beyond what is needed to deliver their core functions. Powerful interest groups will capture increasing portions of resources. Institutional rigidities develop which reduce economic growth.[42] This analysis has led

---

Box 10.2: High Powered Incentives of Ownership[40]

Suppose a transaction involves several people supplying labor, physical inputs, etc. If all but one of the parties involved have contracted to receive fixed amounts, then there is only one residual claimant. In that case, maximizing the value received by the residual claimant is the same as maximizing the total value received by all parties. If the residual claimant also has residual control then just by pursuing his own interests and maximizing his own returns the claimant will be led to make efficient decisions. The combination of residual control and residual claims provides strong incentives and capacity for an owner to maintain and increase an assets value. Firms often attempt to reproduce these high-powered incentives by allocating residual claims in the form of bonuses or shares to key decision-makers in their firm. Misalignment of residual rights and returns causes serious problems. The residual claimant to the returns from a state-owned enterprises is the public purse, but the residual decision-makers are effectively the enterprise manager, the workers, and the bureaucrats in the supervising ministry. None of these has any great personal stake in the value of the enterprise. The resulting low productivity is well documented. Another example of misalignment comes from the U.S. Savings and Loan industry. Those who had the right to control the S&L's investment also had the right to keep any profits earned but were not obligated to make good on losses. That combination of rights and obligations created an incentive for risk taking and fraud what was not effectively countered by other devices during most of the 1980s.[41]

These fields of analysis have led to better understanding of the institutional sources of government failure. The framework has been used to design organizational reforms which seek to allocate to the holders of critical information the authority to make relevant decisions and the financial incentive to do so (in the form of residual claims on the outcome of the decision).

---

public choice theorists to support conservative political agendas (minimizing the role of the state).

Below we discuss how these insights on incentives, contracting, and governance have influenced recent reforms in health service delivery.

A New Model for Private Participation

The degree of public and private involvement in the health sector is rarely strongly influenced by technical or systemic analysis alone. Rather, in the real world, service delivery arrangements are the product of complex economic, institutional, and political factors.

Extensive reforms of public sector organizations and state-owned enterprises have been implemented in the past 15 years to address the very same problems exhibited in public health service provision. Based on a realization that the problems exhibited by the organizations were structural in nature and using the analytical tools of organizational economics, these reforms have focused on altering the institutional arrangements for service. It is worth reviewing these developments, since they shed some light on similar problems found in public delivery of health services.

One way to understand organizational reforms in service delivery is to view the different incentive environments within which the tasks of government can be performed (see Figure 10.4).[43] The civil or core public service lies at the center (usually constitutional control bodies, line ministries), and the activities of the staff are highly determined. Job tenure is also quite strong. Budgetary units (government departments), autonomous units, corporatized units and privatized units are four common organizational modalities that straddle these incentive environments in the health sector.[44]

Figure 10.4
Incentive Environments

Markets/Private
Sector

Broader Public Sector

Core Public Sector

B   A   C   P

B - Budgetary Units
A - Autonomous Units
C - Corporatized Units
P - Privatized Units

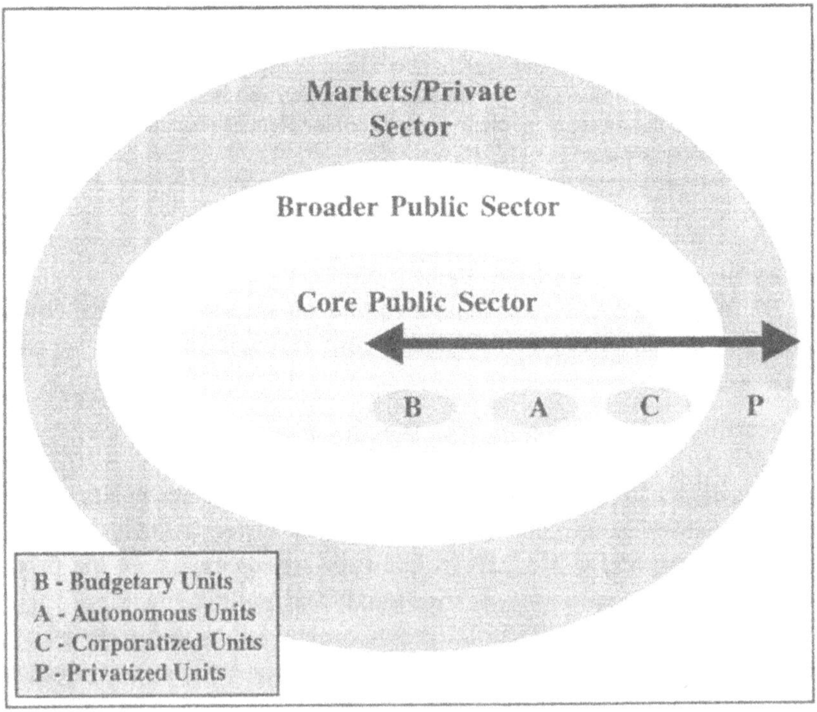

The broader public sector is distinguished by the relative flexibility of the financial management regime, and greater freedom to managers in recruitment and promotion. This may include special purpose agencies, autonomous agencies, and on the outer limits state-owned enterprises. Beyond the public sector lies the domain of the market and civil society. Services may be delivered by for-profit, non-profit or community organizations. The incentives for efficient production are higher as you move out, and service delivery is often better here.

Many reforms throughout the world have sought to move delivery away from the center of the circle to more arm's length contracts with public and private sector organizations. However, there are constraints to moving delivery outward related to the nature of the outputs and the existence of mechanisms for public sector management of their delivery.

Increased autonomy or corporatization—moving from the center of the circle to the outer limits—requires accountability mechanisms not tied to direct control. These controls, such as contracts, take considerable capacity to write and enforce, especially for services in the case of health services where outputs and outcomes are difficult to specify precisely.

How far countries may go in pushing activities to incentive environments in the outer circles depends on the nature of the outputs (the services involved) and the capacity to create accountability for public objectives through indirect mechanisms such as regulation and contracting.

The following section develops several models for mapping public and private health services into these incentive environments based on empirical evidence and recent economic, institutional, and political theories.

Nature of Goods Based on Neoclassical Economics

The model still used most frequently by mainstream economists—yet perhaps least helpful for understanding the optimal mix in public and private involvement in the health sector—is based on a breakdown of the nature of health care goods and service as private, mixed or public goods.

According to this approach, private goods exhibit excludability (consumption by one individual prevents consumption by another—

no positive or negative externalities), rivalness (there is competition among goods based on price), and rejectability (individuals can choose to forgo consumption). True public goods have significant elements of non-excludability, non-rivalness, and non-rejectability. Mixed goods have some but not all of the characteristics of private goods (see Figure 10.5).

This theory indicates that a breakdown occurs in both efficiency and equity when public goods or goods with significant externalities are allocated through competitive markets.[45] In fact, by definition, public goods cannot be sold in private markets, thereby creating a strong justification for collective action. Likewise, significant problems occur in efficiency and equity when private good are produced or provided by the public sector.

In reality few health care activities fall under the category of pure public goods. Hospital services and expensive diagnostic and therapeutic care, although often provided through publicly owned facilities at highly subsidized rates, are really private goods and hence marketable. Likewise, ambulatory and long-term residential care, are usually treated as private goods even in highly centrally controlled health care systems because it was difficult, if not impossible, to prevent their sale in the informal economy.

Even many public health activities, such as sanitation services, control and prevention of communicable diseases, health promo-

Figure 10.5
The Nature of Goods Based on Public Economies

	Nature of Economic Good		
Properties	Public	Mixed	Private
Excludability	—	±	+
Rivalry	—	±	+
Rejectability	—	±	+

Consumer Protection	Consumer Goods
Policymaking	Medical Clinics
Regualtions	Hospitals
Setting Standards	Medical Suppliers
Quality Control	Pharmaceuticals

tion, and other activities, such as research and professional education, that generate significant externalities, are not pure public goods. All of these activities have some degree of excludability, rejectability, and rivalness. For example, a vaccine given to one patient cannot simultaneously be consumed by another patient. At will, patients can choose not to be vaccinated. And vaccination programs may compete with each other for market share.

Recently, water and sanitation systems, immunizations programs, public health campaigns, research funding, and postgraduate training have all been provided successfully through the private sector.

A service delivery model of goods characteristics based on neo-classical economics is therefore not helpful in answering two critical questions often asked by policymakers in relation to the reform health systems:

- When is government provision of goods and services directly through publicly owned organizations an appropriate choice?

- Which sector public or private should finance the service and what charges, if any, should be made to patients?

Theory and experience therefore demonstrate that consumption characteristics alone almost never indicate anything about the specific production processes that ensure technical efficiency. Although normative public economics (neo classical) framework is a robust test for justifying the role of public finance or more appropriately, justifying the need for "steering," it does not help us understand the optimal institutional arrangements for service production. The production characteristics (contestability and information asymmetry/measurability) tell us more about.

Nature of Goods Based on Organizational Economics

The principles of institutional economics lead to a much more refined and useful model for understanding the different kinds of institutional arrangements that are required for efficient and effective "rowing."[46] A model along these lines can be developed based on three different and often ignored goods characteristics—contestability, measurability and information asymmetry.

A market can be said to be perfectly contestable if firms can enter it freely (without any resistance from existing firms) and then exit without losing any of their investments, while having equal access to technology (no asset specificity).[47] Contestability allows competition for the market to substitute for competition in the market.

Contestable goods are characterized by low barriers to entry and exit from the market, whereas non-contestable goods have high barriers such as sunk cost, monopoly market power, geographic advantages, and asset specificity. Investments in specific assets represent a "sunk cost" since its value cannot be recovered elsewhere.[48] Two specific assets that are especially relevant in the health sector are expertise and reputation. Once incumbents have invested in activities that result in expertise or generate trust, they enjoy a significant barrier to entry for other potential suppliers, thereby lowering the degree of contestability. Opportunism, on the other hand, will lower such trust or barriers to entry.

Information asymmetry is the degree to which information about the performance of a given activity is available to users, beneficiaries, or contracting purchasing agencies (see earlier discussion under government failure).

Measurability in the health sector, as in other sectors, is the precision with which inputs, processes, outputs, and outcomes of a given good or services can be measured. By definition, it is difficult to measure with a high degree of precision the output and outcome of health services that is characterized by a high degree of information asymmetry.

Application of Model to Health Sector

Applying these often ignored goods characteristics based on the economics of organizations to the health sector produces some interesting but very different results from those described in the previous model (see Figure 10.6). Using this framework, it is possible to categorize services in a matrix along a continuum from high contestability and high measurability (Type I) through to services with low contestability, low measurability, and significant information asymmetry (Type IX). This framework is particularly instructive in helping policymakers think through "make or buy decisions" regarding when the public sector should produce services to achieve sectoral objectives and when they could use indirect mechanisms such as contracting and regulation to influence outcomes.

The retailing of drugs, medical supplies, and other consumables would be the best example of highly contestable goods where outputs are also easy to measure (Type I). There are usually many companies that jostle for a share of the market and few barriers to entry (the initial investment capital is modest and there are few requirements for specialized licensing or skills).

As we move across the first row (Type I to Type III) a number of factors begin contributing to the increasing barriers to entry that are observed, thereby reducing the contestability of the goods or services in question. In the case of the retail of medical drugs, the specialized training/licensing of pharmacists and professional protectionism create moderate barriers to entry (Type II). For different reasons, the wholesale of drugs, medical supplies, and medical equipment has some barrier to entry because of the larger investment requirements and more limited supply and distribution chains (Type II).

Finally, some activities benefit from economies of scale. Once we move across to the Type III category, therefore, the barriers to entry in the case of the production of pharmaceuticals and medical equipment are much higher due to the need for large up-front sunk-costs, and lead-time for research, development and registration of new prod-

Figure 10.6
The Nature of Health Care Goods Based on Organizational Economics

	High Contestability	Medium Contestability	Low Contestability

High Measurability	Type I
	• Retail of
	  • Drugs
	  • Medical Supplies
	  • Other Goods
		Type II
		• Wholesale
		  • Drugs
		  • Medical Supplies
		  • Other Goods
			Type III
			• Production
			  • Pharmaceuticals
			  • High Technology

Meduim Measurability	Type IV • Routine Diagnostics • Hospital Supoort Services • Training	Type V • Management Services	Type VI • High Tech Diagnostics • Research

Low Measurability	Type VII
	• Ambulatory Clinacal Care
	  • Medical
	  • Nursing
	  • Dental
		Type VIII
		• Generals Hospitals
		• Public Health Services
		• Health Insurace
			Type IX
			• Policymaking
			• Monitoring/Evaluation

ucts. Other barriers to entry under this category include product differentiation (specialized medical equipment) and copyright protection (brand-name drugs). In both Type II and III categories, measurability of outputs remains high and there is little information asymmetry.

As we move to the next row (Type IV to Type VI), measurability of the outputs and outcomes become more problematic. Although routine ambulatory diagnostic clinics and hospital support services may be highly contestable (many players in a competitive market with few barriers to entry), monitoring their performance in terms of effectiveness and quality of the services provided is much harder (Type IV). Hospitals that contract out their diagnostic services need to find a way to monitor the results provided by private laboratories. Getting value for money from out-sourced non clinical support services requires skilled contract management.[49]

As we move across to the Type V category, contestability is reduced by various barriers to entry. One cost disadvantage in the case of management services and training would be the learning cure and highly specialized staff requirement, giving existing players a marked advantage over new entrants.

Contestability is even lower when we move to the (Type VI) category. The large up-front sunk-cost requirements and specialized skills needed to undertake activities such as high technology diagnostics or medical research create serious barriers to entry for new players in the market. A further barrier to entry for these activities would be government policies that control or restrict the introduction of some new technologies (CAT or NMR Scanners).

In addition to difficulties in measuring output and outcomes, most clinical services are characterized by an additional constraint of information asymmetry. These services, therefore, belong under the Type VI to Type IX categories, depending on the degree of barrier to entry of the service in question.

At times, information may be readily apparent to patients (e.g., the quality of hotel services such as courtesy of clinical staff, the length of waiting periods, the cleanliness of the bed sheets, the taste of food, and privacy. Without survey techniques, however, such information may not be readily available to the contracting policy makers or administrative staff. At other times, information may be more readily available to clinical staff than patients (e.g., the diagnosis of rare conditions and probability of surviving an operation) or contracting policy makers and administrative staff (e.g., the cost of services).

For these reasons, ambulatory clinical services would fall under the Type VI category (relatively low barriers to entry other than professional qualifications/certification of staff) but high information asymmetry and difficulties measuring outcomes. General hospitals (barriers due to specialization and cost), public health services (barriers due to specialization and crowding out by government production), and health insurance (barriers due to market distortion caused by severe information asymmetry) would fall under the Type VII category.

This leaves very few clear-cut activities such as policymaking, monitoring and evaluation under the Type IX category. The contestability and monitorability of these activities is extremely low.

As described earlier, governments have at their disposal a variety of instruments that they can use to address market imperfections. From least to most intrusive, these include requiring information disclosure, introducing regulations, contracting for services, direct financing or providing subsidies, and public production.

For some goods and services, there are few serious problems related to market failure. In contestable markets, even if there are only a few or one firm present, anti-trust or regulatory attention may be unnecessary. Indeed the cost of such action would be undesirable from efficiency reasons.

In these cases, the only government policies that are needed are those that ensure information disclosure so that patients and others may make informed choices about the goods and services they will purchase (see Figure 10.7).

Most clinical services—such as hospitals and clinics, training, research, public health and health insurance—have some degree of market failure that reduces contestability and measurability. The very nature of services in the health sector allows firms to erect a number of barriers to entry and encourages firms to control their supply and demand chains, making it difficult for competitors to enter the market. Other commonly occurring barriers to entry include sunk costs due to economies of scale, collusion (e.g., price setting), specialization, and encouraging governments to introduce polices that are favorable to the firm in question but which place a restriction on the

Figure 10.7
Policies to Deal with Reduced Contestability and Measurability

	High Contestability	Medium Contestability	Low Contestability
High Measurability	Information Disclosure		
Meduim Measurability		Regulations and Contracting	
Low Measurability			Public Financing Production

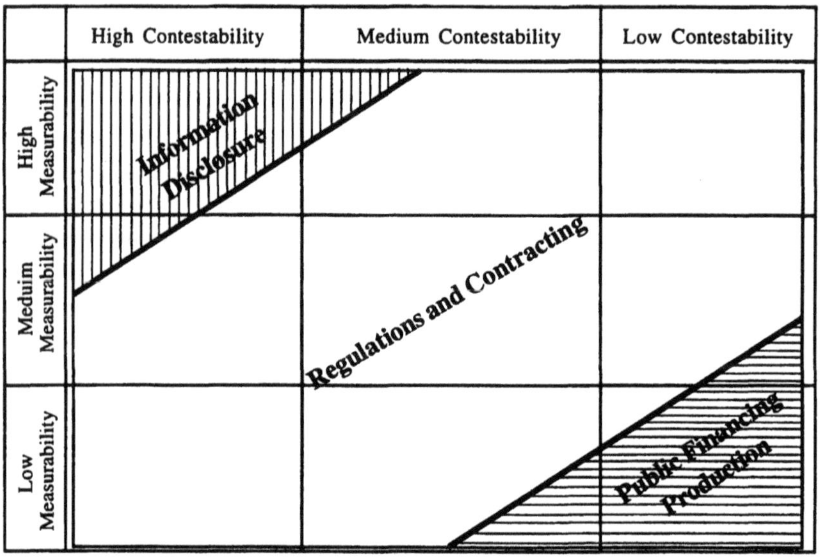

free exit and entry by others (e.g., patent laws and specialist certification).

Despite this complex landscape in goods characteristics, in many areas of reduced contestability and measurability, governments could achieve most equity, efficiency and quality objectives through regulations and contracting.[50]

Instead, in many countries governments have chosen to address this middle band of medium to low contestability and measurability through direct in-house production that would be best reserved for areas of more severe market distortions such as financing. Many of resulting services are fraught with the government failure problems discussed earlier.

Policy Levers Available to Governments

The nature of health care goods and services with respect to contestability/measurability—is not static but rather is influenced by elements of the systemic environment. Government policies directly influence this environment and the "nature of the good" yielding alternative levers to take them closer (or further) away from the ability to use the indirect tools of contracting and regulation (see Figure 10.8). These alternative levers include:

● Governance: Alternating the relationship between governments and health care organizations (governance or internal incentive regime);

● Market environment: Increasing the level of competition in the markets for the relevant goods or services; and

● Purchasing mechanisms: Changing the funding or payments arrangements for the goods or services.

These three factors exert a powerful influence on the nature of the goods" and hence on the ability to ensure delivery through indirect mechanisms. In the next three sections, we will discuss how these factors combine to determine the level of contestability in the market or measurability of a good. This will include a discussion of which instruments are effective in dealing with the related market and government failures.

Governance and Internal Incentive Regime

Changes made in the relationship between government and organizations—governance—influence the goods characteristics of the

Figure 10.8
Key Determinants of Changes in Goods Characteristics

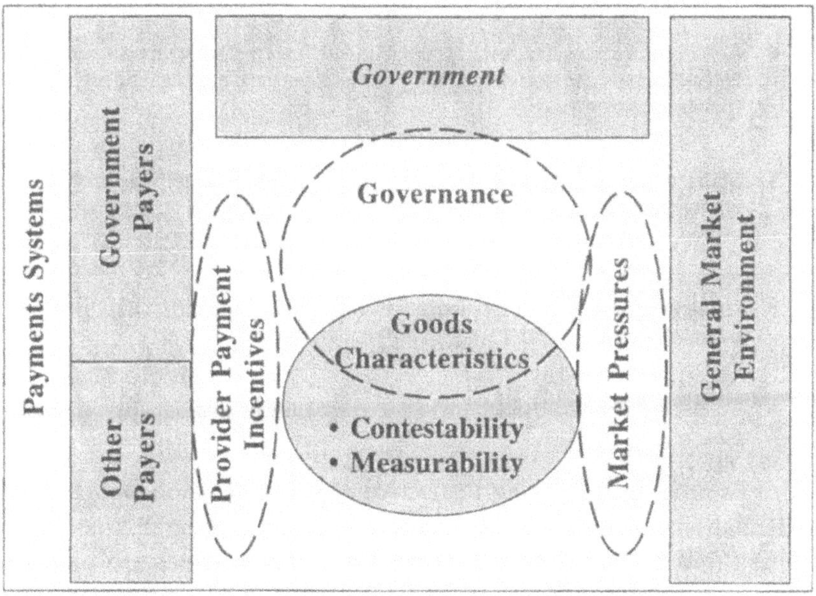

health care goods and services in question. This relationship can be modified substantially in five different dimensions: (a) the decision rights managers are given; (b) the residual claimant status; (c) the degree of market exposure; (d) accountability arrangements; and (e) adequacy of subsidies to cover social functions (see Box 10.3).[51]

Organizational reforms that alter these five critical elements of the internal incentive regime can alter the contestability and measurability of the goods and services in question.

Contestability may be enhanced by:

- Unbundling of large bureaucratic structures (governance)

- Outsourcing other functions to specialized providers (payments)

- Leveling the playing field by exposing all the actors (public and private) to the same potential benefits and losses due to market exposure (governance/payments)

- Decreasing barriers to entry due to political interference or unwarranted trust in public production (market)

- Explicitly separating contestable commercial functions and non-commercial social objectives (governance)

Measurability may be enhanced by:

- Relying on quantifiable results (output or outcomes measures) for accountability and performance targets rather than process (inputs and bureaucratic procedures) (payments, governance?)

- Shifting from difficult to define long-term relationships (employment or service arrangements) to shorter-term and more specific contractual arrangements (payments)

- Using quantifiable monetary incentives rather than more difficult to track non-monetary incentives (ethics, ethos, and status) payments

- Tightening reporting, monitoring and accountability mechanisms (payments/governance)

For example, by removing restrictive government monopolies from vaccination services (governance/market), such programs could be shifted into a Type II or even Type I position. It is easy to measure the number of children vaccinated or who contracted a given disease and moderately low barriers to entry for firms that wanted to provide such services on behalf of the government. Similar action

---

Box 10.3: Five Critical Elements of Internal Incentive Regime

Organizational reforms that alter the goods characteristics of health care goods and services can be characterized by five critical changes in their internal incentive regime (see Figure 10.9 below).

First, decision rights can be shifted from the hierarchy—or supervising agency—to the organization itself. Critical decision rights transferred to management may include control over: inputs, labor, scope of activities, financial management, clinical and non-clinical administration, strategic management (formulation of institutional objectives), market strategy, and sales.

Second, managers and staff can be given strong financial incentives to economize by making them rather than the public purse the "residual claimant" on revenue flows—giving them the right to keep retained earnings and the proceeds from the sale of capital. "Why scrimp and save if you cannot keep the results of your frugality?"[52] Aligning the revenue flows with decision rights in this way can have a powerful impact on the behavior of the organization.

Third, the degree to which revenues are earned in a market rather than through a direct budget allocation is another high powered incentive that can be introduced through organizational reforms. If delivering quality services to patients is the best way to generate revenue, then that strategy will be pursued. On the other hand, if political lobbying, or extracting monopoly rents is the best way to get revenue, then these strategies will be pursued.

Fourth, as decision-rights are delegated to the organization, the ability by governments to assert direct accountability (through the hierarchy) is diminished. But markets are not capable of delivering the full range of sectoral objectives both due to market failures and due to social values. Accountability under the new arrangement can still be secured by shifting from hierarchical supervision to reliance on regulations or the economic incentives imbedded in contracts.[53]

The fifth critical factor characterizing organizational reforms is the degree to which "social functions" delivered by organizations are shifted from being implicit and unfunded to specified and directly funded. As organizations are encouraged to focus more on financial viability, due to the changes discussed above, management will move to decrease output of services that don't cover their costs. Maintaining a financial bottom line, therefore, undermines the ability to cross-subsidize certain services internally. To preserve equity and avoid adverse selection, alternative measures must be introduced to ensure that services, which were previously cross-subsidized, continue to be delivered for low income and other vulnerable populations.

applied to other services could shift many away from the lower right corner of the grill towards the upper left corner (see Figure 10.9).

Likewise, through better information on outcome and policies that favored clearly defined contracts, performance benchmarks, and a tightening of reporting, monitoring and accountability mechanisms, and tertiary and quaternary care provided in university hospitals could be shifted from a low contestability/measurability grid to a medium contestability/measurability position.

Several factors may also alter the goods characteristics of pharmaceuticals, medical equipment, and consumable supplies.

Medical equipment or drugs that were highly specialized and very expensive due to development costs, patent protection, and a small market share (Type III goods) as little as 10 year ago, may today behave as ordinary goods (Type II or I). Examples include the quick production of generic drugs by many companies once patent protection expires or the rapid increase in use of sigmoidoscopes and or transcutaneous surgical instruments once the technology is no longer new and prices have dropped.

Figure 10.9
The Nature of Health Care Goods Based on Organizational Economics

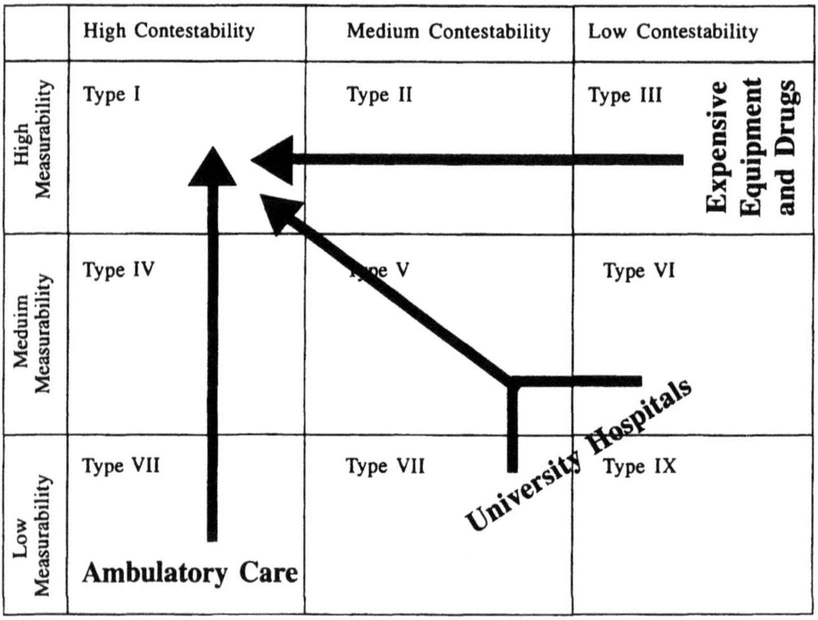

	High Contestability	Medium Contestability	Low Contestability
High Measurability	Type I	Type II	Type III Expensive Equipment and Drugs
Meduim Measurability	Type IV	Type V	Type VI
Low Measurability	Type VII Ambulatory Care	Type VII	Type IX University Hospitals

Because of these factors, health care goods and services may drift across the contestability/measurability grid in a more dynamic way that would be indicated in the earlier static model, once barriers to entry in terms of required sunk cost and other restrictions disappear.

This shift in goods characteristics is not a one-way street. The goods properties can also become less contestable and more difficult to measure. Organizational reforms do not always lead to increased decision rights, residual claimant status, market exposure, accountability arrangements and explicit subsidies to cover social functions. In fact, during the past 50 years, many of the national health systems that were introduced through a nationalization of ownership and production deliberately shifted goods and services in the opposite direction.

And market imperfections, may contribute to rather than lower barriers to entry. Doctors, dentists and pharmacists can and do collude to restrict entry by potential competitors. Hospitals have a natural monopoly for their services for patients living nearby, and can create monopoly power through relations with other hospitals and referring doctors. Medical equipment distributors with licensing agreements for the top international companies can easily monopolize a domestic market. Pharmaceutical retailers can control their mark-up through formation of professional cartels. The public and non-governmental sectors have a competitive advantage over the private sector due to their access to subsidized or free capital from domestic and foreign donors.

The next section deals with the systemic measures—competitive environment and provider payment mechanisms—that can be to put into place to further enhance contestability and measurability.

Competitive Environment

One of the central arguments in favor of exposing providers to market forces is that in a functioning market, competitive forces will lead to a more efficient allocation of resources than command economy or non-market solutions. The structure of the market to which organizations are exposed, therefore, has a critical influence on their behavior. It may directly determine what strategies will make sense to generate more revenue.

Policies that influence the competitive environment through regulations or contracting can significantly alter the contestability of health care goods and services. Likewise, policies that increase the availability of good information on health services, that enhance the institutional capacity by health care providers to deal with such information, and that improve patients' understanding about health problems, can reduce information asymmetry.

Such policies not only address some of the underlying contestability and measurability problems, but they actually shift both the contestability/measurability grid and the boundaries of needed government intervention to ensure favorable outcomes (see Figure 10.10).

Conversely, in a less competitive environment with weak policies and data to overcome information asymmetry, the grid for services that fall into the upper left corner (Types I, II, and IV) may contract with the grid in the lower right corner (VI, VIII, and IX) expanding. Some examples of this will be given below.

Market Imperfections in Service Delivery

There are two related problems in the market structure of service delivery in most segments of the health sector. First, little or no com-

Figure 10.10
Shifting the Contestability/Measurability Grid and Needed Public Policies

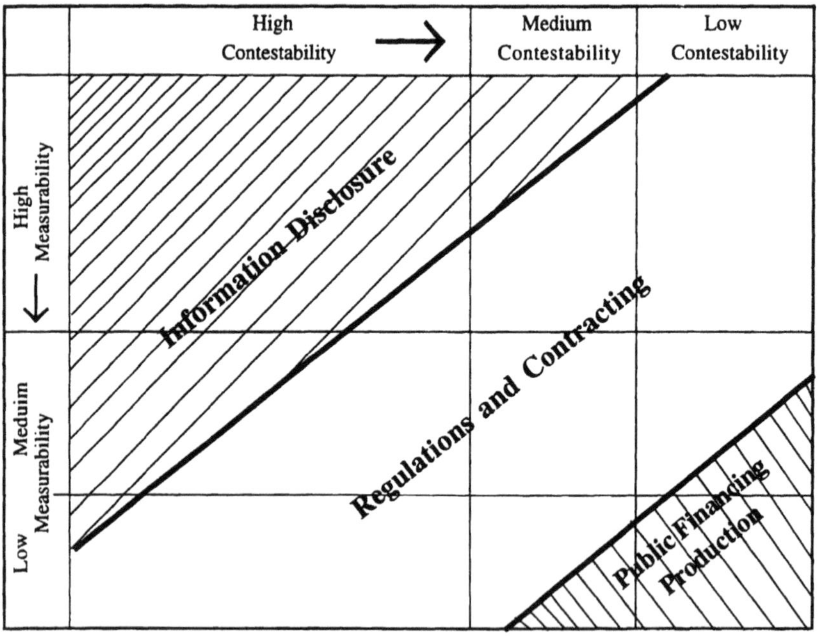

petition may emerge—reducing the pressures on the provider to deliver "value for money" in order to maximize profits. Alternatively (or in addition), competition may emerge, but it may be dysfunctional. Both cases are discussed in this section.

Some health services especially tertiary and quaternary, exhibit scale economies in production. This relieves incumbent hospitals from pressure from new entrants. Geographic monopoly over certain services may leave buyers with very little leverage in negotiating with service providers. There are many examples of strong collusion among medical doctors to create a virtual monopoly, thereby shifting the grid for ambulatory medical care towards the left-and strengthening the need for direct provision or other policy intervention. Public monopolies and policies that prevent public funds from being used to contract services from the private sector have the same negative effect on contestability.

Even for services where monopoly power is not an issue, providers may still capture market share or maximize profits through various forms of distortionary behavior (see Figure 10.11).

Figure 10.11
Market Forces That Influence Competition

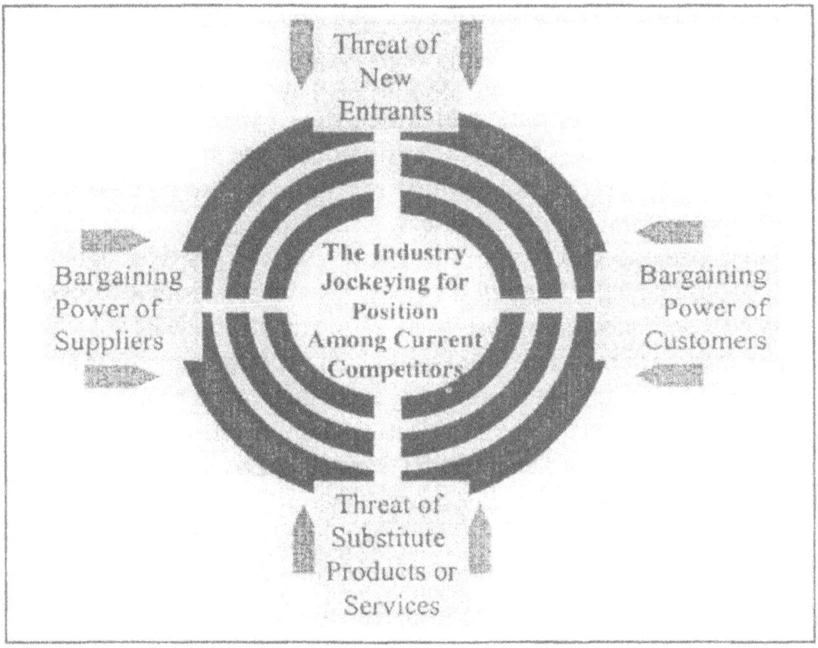

In a competitive market, firms seek to maximize their profits and they seek to do so using whichever method makes sense in that environment. In a healthy market environment, they will try to capture market share from their competitors by better pleasing customers, to maximize profits by reducing costs through efficiency gains, and to expand their product lines through imitation or innovation. Wherever possible, however, they will seek to exploit or construct advantages. Where this is possible, the pressures for efficiency and quality generated by the market may be very weak.

Such distortionary features of health service markets often give providers the ability to: (a) counter the bargaining power of suppliers, patients or purchasers; (b) ward off the threats posed by new entrants and imitation products; and (c) control a large share of relevant market.

The information asymmetry that exists in the health sector exacerbates these problems. For example, medical treatment is to a large extent a "bundled" good where the seller (doctor) is guiding patients' consumption decisions—which hospital to go to for surgery, which lab to use for diagnostic services, and so on. Thus, the providers' information advantage can be parlayed into control over a rigid and lucrative referral chain. Doctors may "forward integrate" into diagnostic labs, or pharmacies and steer their patients toward consumption where they have a financial stake. Hospitals may "backward integrate" by creating strong links with doctors, thereby creating a portion of the market in which they experience little or no competitive pressure. Medical professionals are frequently able to create cartels, limiting competitive pressures that strengthen the influence of patients and purchasers.

Since patients and payers know less than the provider about the true value or cost of health services, providers are able to cream-skim or select patients whose costs of treatment are relatively lower than other patients. Thus, providers can increase their profits not through delivering better services to capture market share, or cutting costs, but rather through selecting more profitable patients.

Most of these market imperfections in service delivery can be corrected through appropriate regulations and contracting arrangements.

A few examples will illustrate this point. Anti-trust legislation, limiting the power of professional cartels and availability of equal access to capital can significantly decrease the barrier to entry for some segments of the health care market, especially in the case of the clinical services that fall in the middle band of the contestability/measurability grid. The same would be true for contracting practices that are open to both the public and private sector providers, and that leave open the possibilities of which create the possibility of choosing alternative providers or exercising "exit" strategies.

There are other instances where supplier cartels combined with low quality control standards shift activities such as the retail and distribution of pharmaceuticals and medical equipment into the lower right corner, even though such activities belong in the upper left area of high contestability and measurability.

Market imperfections of private health insurance. Even if private health insurance is contestable, due to severe information asymmetry, such services are often deliberately crowded out for strategic reasons by restrictive policies and public financing. This topic is beyond the scope of the discussion presented in this chapter but discussed in detail elsewhere (see Box 10.4).[54]

Box 10.4
The Intractable Market Imperfections of Private Health Insurance

Private voluntary health insurance is one area that is particularly prone to a number of market imperfections, many of which relate to information asymmetries. While insurance may succeed in protecting some people against selected risks, it usually fails to cover everyone willing to subscribe to insurance plans and it often excludes those who need health insurance the most or who are at greatest risk of illness. This happens because insurers have a strong incentive to enroll only healthy or low-cost clients (risk selection or cream-skimming). Private insurers also have incentives to exclude costly conditions or to minimize their financial risk through the use of benefit caps and exclusions. This limits protection against expensive/catastrophic illnesses.

Because of these factors, individuals who know they are at risk of illness have a strong incentive to conceal their underlying medical condition (adverse selection). Individuals who are-or at least think they are-healthy will often try to pay as low premiums as possible. This prevents insurers from raising the funds needed to cover the expenses incurred by sicker or riskier members. Worse, the healthy may even deliberately under-insure themselves, in the hope that free or highly subsidized care will be available when they become ill (free-riding). When third-party insurers pay, both patients and providers have less incentive to be concerned about costs, and some may even become careless about maintaining good health. This leads not only to more care being used (the reason for insurance), but also to less effective care, or care that would not be needed if people maintained good health (moral hazard).

Provider Payment Systems

Provider payment systems also influence goods properties by interacting with three of the five key elements of the internal incentive regime of health care organizations: distribution of residual claims, market exposure and provisions for social functions.

While reforms in governance may endow a given organization with formal claims to residual revenue in different categories, the structure of the payments system will directly determine whether this claim has any real meaning or incentive effect. If, for example, services must be delivered at prices less than cost, there will be no residual to claim. Thus the relationship of costs to the price setting and capital charging formula in the payments system is a critical determinant of the incentives of the model. The crucial factor is whether marginal cost saving effort on the part of the provider can generate revenue flows that the provider can keep.

When reforms to an organization hospital entail a shift to earning its revenue through delivering services "in a market," the issue of what kind of market actually emerges becomes crucial. Often the government is the largest, or only buyer. In this case, the process and terms on which the government purchaser engages the provider may well determine the degree of pressure they are under to "deliver the goods."

To gain maximum benefits from reforms that expose the public sector to competition with the private sector, it is crucial that adequate steps are taken to secure competitive neutrality. Two sets of policies must be built into provider payment systems to achieve this:

- Moneterization of social functions (explicit subsidies that adequately cover the cost plus a reasonable margin in delivering services to non-paying or non-insured patients)

- Leveling of the playing field through a standardization of the fee structure and cost of capital for both the public and private sector.

For example, as managers start to cost their activities, the (prices set in the) payment system will determine which services cover their costs (for services which are purchased by the government). They will reduce internal cross subsidization where possible. If the organizations have been playing a substantial safety net role, by generating funds from some services to cover costs of services delivered to needy portions of the population, then the payments system will need to take this into account. The government's choices regarding which services (or which patients) to subsidize will determine the degree to which unfunded mandates requiring internal cross subsidization lead to adverse selection and exclusion of poorer patients.

Likewise, without policies that level the playing field, the public and non-governmental sectors will have a distinct competitive advantage due to their access to subsidized or free capital. Differential fee or contract structures are designed to include a capital allowance that compensates for such imbalances.

Conclusions

The health sector is fraught with both market and government production failure.

This chapter has demonstrated the need for an enhanced role of the state in providing strong stewardship in the health sector. But it challenges the principles and nature of public intervention pursued by many governments especially in the area of the public production of health services.

The latter is typically associated with problems in accountability, information asymmetry, abuse of monopoly power, and failure to formulate and execute policies in several areas that are critical in securing better health for the population.

Applying this framework based on recent developments in organizational economics yields a strong case for recourse to the disciplining pressures of competition or exit strategies which come from greater private participation in providing health services as a powerful tool for improving the performance of both public and private health service delivery systems.

In fact, empirical and theoretical evidence suggests that monopolistic public provision is unlikely to ever be the best practice. Rather institutional pluralism (with many players wearing many different hats) is more likely to be at the core of efficient service delivery systems in the future. This will place greater demands on the state and public administration/management to play a more nuanced role in ensuring that pluralistic contractual arrangements are actually mutually binding, credible, and enforceable.

At the same time, the analysis supports a more focused engagement by governments in securing equity, efficiency, and quality

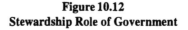

Figure 10.12
Stewardship Role of Government

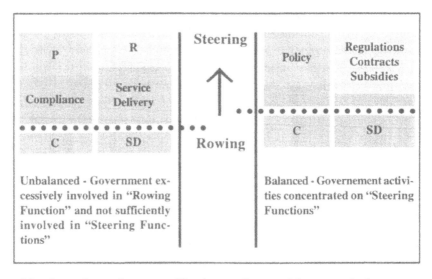

objectives through more effective policy making, regulating, contracting, and financing, that is, steering, not rowing (see Figure 10.12).

Notes

1.   The USA, Mexico and Turkey are three exceptions in the OECD where universal access has not yet been secured. For a review of the introduction of universality in the OECD, see Preker, A., *The Introduction of Universality in Health Care*, London: IIHS, 1989.
2.   For a comprehensive review, see Young, P., *Privatization Around the Globe: Lessons from the Reagan Administration*, Houston: National Center for Policy Analysis, January 1986; and Vickers, J.S. and G.K. Yarrow, *Privatization: An Economic Analysis*, Cambridge, MA: MIT Press, 1988.
3.   Barr, N., Ed., *Labor Markets and Social Policy in Central and Eastern Europe*, Oxford: World Bank/Oxford, 1994; and World Bank, Chapter 8, "Investing in People and Growth," in *1996 World Development Report*: From Plan to Market, New York: Oxford University Press, 1996; 123-132.
4.   World Health Organization (WHO), 1999 World Health Report, Geneva: WHO, 1999; World Health Organization, *European Health Care Reforms: Analysis of Current Strategies*, Series No 72, Copenhagen: WHO Regional Office for Europe, 1996; World Bank, 1993 *World Development Report: Investing in Health*, New York: Oxford University Press, 1993; World Bank, *Sector Strategy: Health, Nutrition, and Population*, Washington: World Bank, 1997; and UNICEF, *State of the World's Children*; New York: UNICEF, 1999.
5.   For a review of the health care problems in the former socialist states, see Preker A.S., and R.G.A. Feachem, *Market Mechanisms and the Health Sector in Central and Eastern Europe*, Technical Paper Series No. 293, Washington: World Bank, 1996 (translations into Russian, Hungarian, Polish, Romanian and Czech).

6. This functional framework of the health sector is based on a modification of the work by Joseph Kutzin, World Health Organization, Londono, J.-L., and Frenk, J., "Structured pluralism: Towards an innovative model for health system reform in Latin America," *Health Policy*, 41 (1997), 1-36.

7. Most health economists—even those favoring a more competitive marketplace—recognize that government needs to play a significant role in the health sector. For an excellent recent review on this topic see Rice, T., *The Economics of Health Reconsidered*, Chicago: Health Administration Press, 1998.

8. We will only map health care financing in general terms into the overall framework presented in this chapter. For a more detailed discussion on the theory and empirical evidence of public and private roles in health care financing see Musgrove, P., *Public and Private Roles in Health: Theory and Financing Patterns*, Washington: World Bank, 1996; and Schieber, G., (ed), *Innovations in Health Financing*, Washington: World Bank, 1996.

9. One of the first proposals for this approach was published by Enthoven, A., "Consumer Choice Health Plan," *The New England Journal of Medicine*, 298(12): 650-58 and 298(13): 709-20 (1978); Enthoven, A., *Theory and Practice of Managed Competition in Health Care Finance*, Netherlands: North-Holland, 1988.

10. See Rice, Op. Cit, 1998.

11. For a comprehensive discussion, see Evans, R.G., Strained Mercy, Toronto: Butterworth, 1984. The classics include: Bator, F., "The Anatomy of Market Failure," *Quarterly Journal of Economics*, 72 (1958); Atkinson, A.B., and J.E. Stiglitz, Lectures on Public Economics, Maidenhead: McGraw-Hill, 1980; and Musgrave, R.A. and P.B. Musgrave, *Public Finance in Theory and Practice*, 4th edition, New York: McGraw-Hill, 1984.

12. For a more comprehensive discussion, see Barer, Morris, L., Thomas E. Getzen and Greg L. Stoddart (Eds.), *Health, Health Care and Health Economics: Perspectives on Distribution*, Chichester, West Sussex, England: John Wiley & Sons, 1998; and van Doorslaer, E., A. Wagstaff, and F. Rutten, Eds., *Equity in the Finance and Delivery of Health Care: An International Perspective*, Oxford: Oxford Medical Publications, 1993. The classical reference is Arrow, K. W., "Uncertainty and the Welfare Economics of Medical Care," *American Economics Review*, 53(5), 1963: 940-73.

13. See Musgrove, Op. Cit, 1996.

14. This topology of the public and private mix in health care financing and service delivery is based on concepts first developed by Reinhardt, U.E., "The U.S. Health Care Financing and Delivery System: Its Experience and Lessons for Other Nations," *International Symposium on Health Care Systems*, December 18-19, 1988.

15. See Osborne, D. , and T. Gaebler, *Reinventing Government*, New York: Plume, 1993.

16. See Saltman, R., and J. Figueras, (Eds.), *European Health Care Reform: Analysis of Current Strategies WHO*, 1997, 213-214.

17. See Wilson, J.Q., *Bureaucracy*, New York: Basic Books, 1989; Donahue, J.D., *The Privatization Decision: Public Ends, Private Means*, New York: Basic Books, 1989; and World Bank, *World Development Report: The State in a Changing World*, New York: Oxford University Press, 1997.

18. Wolf, C.J., "A Theory of Non-Market Failure," *Journal of Law and Economics*, 22:1 (1979), 107-39; Peacock, A, "On the Anatomy of Collective Failure," *Public Finance*, 35:1 (1980), 33-43; Weimer, D.L. and A.R. Vining, *Policy Analysis: Concept and Practice*, Englewood Cliffs: Prentice Hall, 1989; Vining, A.R. and D.L., Weimer, "Government Supply and Government Production Failure: A Framework Based on Contestability," *J. Publ. Pol.*, 10: 1 (1990), 1-22.

19. Much of this discussion is not new but firmly rooted in political and moral. See Arrow, K., *Arrow's Theorem: The Paradox of Social Choice*, New Haven: Yale University, 1980.

20. Although there are no technical limits, few countries like Switzerland use plebiscites, and only for major issues of national interest. Even then it is an imperfect instrument due to low voter turnout.

21. Four interrelated causes have been identified that explain this observation (see Vining, A.R. and D.L., Weimer, "Government Supply and Government Production Failure: A Framework Based on Contestability," *J. Publ. Pol.*, 10: 1 (1990), p. 15.). First, direct democracy usually prevents the overseer from knowing the preferences of society. Second, overseers (representatives) typically pay more attention to those constituencies and sensational issues that are most likely to be influential in their re-election. Third, public officials usually have more than one overseer, often leading to conflicting and unstable political demands. Finally, since overseers do not fully benefit themselves from the effectiveness of their oversight, they often devote inadequate time and effort to this task, leaving bureaucrats with a large range of independence.

22. This conceptual framework was developed by Moore, M., *Creating Public Value*, Boston: Harvard University Press, 1995.

23. We will discuss this further in a later section under agency problems. Beauchamp, T.L., and Childress, J.F. *Principles of Biomedical Ethics*, 2nd ed., Oxford: Oxford University Press, 1983, 4; and Lemmon, E.J., "Moral Dilemmas," *Philosophical Review*, 71 (1962): 139-152.

24. See theoretical section for a more complete discussion of the principal—agent concepts. Bennett, S., McPake, B., and Mills, A. (eds.) *Private Health Providers in Developing Countries: Serving the Public Interest?* London: Zed Books, 1997.

25. Fama, E.F., M.C. Jensen, "Agency Problems and Residual Claims," *Journal of Law and Economics*, 26:2 (1983), 327-49.

26. Kaufmann, D. and R. Ryterman, "Global Corruption Survey," World Bank Working Paper, Washington: World Bank, 1998.

27. Hirschman, A., *Exit, Voice, and Loyalty: Responses to Decline in Firms, Organizations, and States*, Cambridge, MA: Harvard University Press, 1970; World Bank, 1997, Op. Cit.

28. This narrow approach is developed in detail in Rice, Op. Cit., 1998.

29. Named after the economist Vilfredo Pareto.

30. Neoclassical economic theory shows that if certain conditions are met, allowing competition to occur will result in an equilibrium situation where it is impossible to make someone better off without making someone else worse off.

31. See Robinson, J., "Physician-Hospital Integration and Economic Theory of the Firm," in *Medical Care Research and Review*, 54:1 (March 1997).

32. OECD, *Regulatory Reform, Privatisation and Competition Policy*, Paris: OECD, 1992, 17.

33. Sappington, D.E., "Incentives in Principal Agent Relationships," *Journal of Economic Perspectives*, 5:2 (1991), 45-66.

34. Fama, E.F. "Agency Problems and the Theory of the Firm," *Journal of Political Economy*, 88:2 (1980), 288-307; and, Jensen, M. C., W.H. Meckling, "Theory of the Firm: Managerial Behavior, Agency Costs and Ownership Structure," *Journal of Financial Economics*, 3 (1976): 305-60.

35. See Williamson, O., "Comparative Economic Organization: The Analysis of Discrete Structural Alternatives," *Administrative Science Quarterly*, 36 (June 1991), 69-296.

36. Two useful references include: Williamson, O., *The Economic Institutions of Capitalism: Firms, Markets and Relational Contracting*, Free Press, 1985; and Williamson, O., "Transaction Cost Economics," Chapter 3 in Schmalensee, R. and R. Willig, (Eds.), *Handbook of Industrial Economics*, North-Holland, 1989.

37. See Milgrom, P. and J. Roberts "Bargaining Costs, Influence Costs, and the Organization of Economic Activity" in Alt, J., and K. Shepsle, (Eds.), *Perspectives on Positive Political Economy*, Cambridge, 1990.

38. See Milgrom, P. and Roberts, J., *Economics of Organization and Management*, Printice Hall, 1992, Chapter 9.

39. For example, an owner may own a house, but not have the right to occupy it if he has leased it out. He may own a car but not have the right to transfer it freely if he has a loan secured by the car.

40. Milgrom and Roberts, Op. Cit., 1992, 291.

41. Milgrom and Roberts, Op. Cit., 1992, 292.

42. Olson, M., *The Rise and Decline of Nations: Economic Growth, Stagflation and Social Rigidities*, New Haven: Yale University Press, 1982.

43. Adapted from Manning, N., "Unbundling the State: Autonomous Agencies and Service Delivery," Draft World Bank Discussion Paper, 1998.

44. See Harding, A., and A.S. Preker, (Eds.), *Innovations in Health Service Delivery: Corporatization in the Hospital Sector*, New York: Oxford, forthcoming 1999. In other parts of the public sector, such autonomous and corporatized units are also variedly referred to as public or executive agencies, independent public organizations (IPOs), quasi-autonomous non-governmental organizations (QANGOs), and state-owned enterprises (SOEs). There is no standard functional distinction between these different organizational modalities.

45. Musgrove, Op. Cit., 1986; and Evans, Op. Cit., 1984.

46. Girishankar, N., "Reforming Institutions for Service Delivery: A Framework for Development Assistance with an Application to the HNP Portfolio," World Bank Policy Research Working Paper 2039, Washington: World Bank, 1999.

47. Baumol, W.J., J.C. Panzar, and R.D. Willing, *Contestable Markets and the Theory of Industrial Structure*, New York: Harcourt Brace Jovanovich, 1982; and Baumol, W.J. "Towards a Theory of Public Enterprise," *Atlantic Economic Journal*, 12:1 (1984), 3-20. For a critique of this theory, see W.G. Shepherd, "Contestability vs. Competition-Once More," *Land Economics*, 71:3 (August 1995), 299-309; and W.G. Shepherd, "Contestability vs. Competition," 74:4 (1984), 572-587.

48. An asset is specific if it makes a much larger contribution to the production of a good than its value in alternative uses. See Klein, B., R.G. Crawford, and A.A. Alchian, "Vertical Integration, Appropriable Rents and the Competitive Contracting Process," *Journal of Law and Economics*, 21:2 (1978), 297-26.

49. For a detailed review of the literature on this topic, see Broomberg, J., Mills, A., *Experiences of Contracting: An Overview of the Literature*, Technical Paper No. 33, Macro-economics, Health and Development Series (ICO), Geneva: World Health Organization, 1998; Mills, A. *Improving the Efficiency of Public Sector Health Services in Developing Countries: Bureaucratic versus Market Approaches*, PHP Department Publication No. 17, London: London School of Hygiene and Tropical Medicine, 1995; and Bennett, S., S. Russell, and A. Mills, *Institutional and Economic Perspectives on Government Capacity to Assume New Roles in the Health Sector, A Review of Experience*, PHP Department Publication No. 22, London: London School of Hygiene and Tropical Medicine, 1995.

50. See Herzlinger R.E., *Market Driven Health Care: Who Wins, Who Loses in the Transformation of America's Largest Service Industry*, Reading, MA: Perseus Books, 1997.

51. For a more complete discussion on organizational reforms, see Harding and Preker, Op. Cit., 1999.
52. Wilson, Op, Cit., 1989, 116.
53. See Pauly, M., "Health Systems Ownership: Can Regulation Preserve Community Benefits," *Frontiers of Health Services Management*, Spring 12:3 1996.
54. See Musgrove, Op. Cit., 1986.

11

Mutual Benefit Societies: Solutions in Europe, North Africa, and Latin America

M. Duranton, A. Zouaq, and J. Pilón

Mutual benefit societies are extensively involved in the social protection systems of many countries. Providing health coverage is their main area of action. Whether managing a basic or a supplementary scheme, or both, mutual benefit societies are inextricably involved in access to health care. Hence, the reform of such systems is of very direct relevance to mutual benefit institutions, whatever their level of activity.

In terms of innovation, the solidarity-based approach of mutual benefit societies guarantees the continuance of the mechanisms that lie at the foundation of social security. More often than not, it is they who initiate reform, as they are aware that, faced with economic difficulties, those in government tend to propose solutions that amount to a withdrawal by the state and that, even though the state no longer guarantees the basic forms of social solidarity, there is the risk that fundamental rights in such cases will be threatened. There can be no question of any approach to solving economic difficulties that involves calling into question the theory of the welfare state, whether in whole or in part.

Obviously, the burden of health care expenditure will inevitably increase in all countries worldwide. In most cases, this means posi-

---

This article is composed of contributions provided by M. Duranton, covering the European aspect, A. Zouaq, outlining developments in Morocco, and J. Pilon, focusing on Latin America.

tive social evolution. Access to increased protection for the greatest possible number of people, progress in medical techniques, and increasing life expectancy are definite improvements. At the same time, the economic criteria of competitivity allow no room for unbalanced national budgets and exert pressure to reduce production costs. The most simplistic solution in this case is to leave it to individual initiative to deal with the consequences of these new needs, the cost of which is constantly growing. In most cases, the need is not for the State to stage a massive withdrawal, but to reduce the share of the cost of health care borne by the community. These processes vary widely in degree and in the techniques used in different countries, but they constitute a general trend today.

Reform processes can also include gaining control of new developments and attempting to cover them in a global policy aimed at both promoting public health care and maintaining a tolerable degree of economic equilibrium in terms of national and international criteria. But such approaches can only be made globally and must address all aspects responsible for cost increases and all the actors involved.

Thus, some different form of responsibility sharing can be conceived and, between the extremes of all-state and all-private systems, the organizing principles of mutual benefit societies, which retain the mechanisms of solidarity and citizenship, can be decisive, since they make it possible at once to make dynamic progress in meeting health care needs and to meet the need to accord greater responsibility to all those involved.

Although the role played by mutual benefit societies in most countries is modest, there are already examples in which progress is possible in this direction and has in part been achieved. This chapter does not aim to describe these examples, but rather to focus on some highly specific areas in which mutual benefit-type measures have formed part of innovations in the organization of health systems. These include the role played by mutual benefit societies:

- in France in the introduction of the "referring physician" system,

- in Morocco in the public service in relation to developments in the sickness benefit scheme, and

- in Uruguay.

In France and Morocco, mutual benefit societies have a particular status. Their history is partly shared, and there are many points of similarity. However, in this case France is addressing a problem linked to measures supplementing the basic scheme, whereas Morocco is witnessing the evolution of a basic scheme managed by a mutual benefit association. The example of Uruguay shows how the ideas of mutual benefit brought by European immigrants to Latin America are alive and active. The examples show the degree to which, in different forms, the mutual benefit approach can play an essential role in relation to innovation and reform in health systems.

The Referring Physician Option in France

One element of the reforms initiated in France to improve the management of health expenditure has consisted of encouraging insured persons, for general medical needs, to use the same doctor, who is then responsible for follow-up on illnesses, prevention and referral to specialists. In view of the attachment to freedom of choice of a doctor for the sick, which is firmly rooted in French culture and fiercely defended by the medical profession, the measures proposed have been aimed to encourage rather than coerce. The referring physician responsible for ensuring the continuity and coordination of care can be chosen by the patient for a period of one year, which may be renewed.

The referring physician receives an annual flat-rate fee for each patient, set at the cost of one-and-a-half consultations. The physician thereby undertakes to respect the rules regarding the attainment of objectives for health care expenditure, the standard medical references system (a guide to good practice concerning prescriptions, X-rays and biological examinations, etc.) and to apply the "Referring Physician's Quality Charter."

The charter entails a number of obligations for physicians:

- not to exceed an annual maximum level of activity beyond which the quality of treatment can no longer be ensured;

- to ensure the constant availability and continuity of treatment, which means that the physician must make arrangements to ensure that, outside his or her normal hours of duty, another doctor is available to provide treatment;

- in group practices, the maximum levels can be consolidated;

- under the contract, the referring physician undertakes to apply the charges agreed by the sickness insurance scheme and not to exceed them;

- the physicians undertake to allow patients exemption from advance payments;

- the physicians are required to keep a medical synthesis dossier that includes all useful information concerning the patient's health, as well as the health book distributed by the sickness insurance scheme;

- where equivalent treatment is available (including through the computerized clinical files (DCI)), the physicians undertake to prescribe the least costly medication;

- the physicians also undertake to prescribe generic medication (at least 5 percent of overall prescriptions issued);

- the physicians undertake to participate in prevention campaigns;

- the physicians must offer their patients follow-up examinations appropriate to the detection of illness and its prevention;

- the physicians must also incorporate into their practices the recommendations and standards of the National Agency for Health Accreditation and Evaluation (ANAES);

- the physicians have priority access to vocational training courses, which they undertake to evaluate.

Patients belonging to the system are excused the advance payment of fees; that is, they are not required to pay the portion of the consultation fee that is reimbursed by the basic scheme.

In France the basic scheme reimburses only 65 percent of medical fees, meaning that in order to be fully operational the system has to cover the remaining 35 percent. If it does not, the system of exempting patients from advance payment is largely ineffective, since the doctor then has to claim the portion of the consultation fee that is not reimbursed by the basic scheme. Mutual benefit societies, which in France cover more than half the population, have hence decided to become involved in promoting the referring physician system.

By entering into an agreement with an association of general physicians and with the main sickness insurance fund—that covering salaried employees—the system has ensured that the exemption from advance payment is fully applied for most members of the mutual benefit scheme.

The system could then have become fully operational if other professional associations of doctors had not instigated complaints procedures with administrative bodies, which has resulted in some of the texts and agreements concluded being re-examined. Efforts are being made to put the agreements into an indisputable form, and new versions have been published that do not fundamentally deviate from the spirit of the reform. Fresh efforts are now being made to recruit doctors to the scheme, with joint information campaigns between health insurance funds and mutual benefit societies. Members of the social security scheme and of the mutual benefit societies are also the target of joint information campaigns. In addition, the technical systems agreed between the basic scheme and the mutual benefit association have been better defined and will be finalized with the introduction of the new version of the social security smart card (VITALE 2).

Whether for specific files such as those kept by the referring physician, or in other areas (implementation of the social security health data network), the basic schemes and associations supplementing them—particularly the mutual benefit societies—have a growing interest in ensuring that their activities are effectively coordinated. Any measures intended to improve the health system will be efficient only if there is coordinated action among those financing it. On the basis of a general protocol agreement, the French mutual benefit societies and the National Health Insurance Fund are hence now working on a health care package involving the possible coordination of the reimbursement policy, thereby preventing cost-control exercises from being nullified by the effects of transferred costs, which have been common in the cost-reduction programs of the basic health insurance schemes over the years.

In order to preserve the solidarity basis of social protection in France, now more than ever before such policies must succeed in achieving their full potential if they are to prevent the notion of a "health care market" from opening the way for purely commercial interests. Whether in ensuring responsible public health policy or preserving equal access for all to good quality health care, political decision-makers must promote this joint venture. The rules of competition cannot be allowed to play the role of regulator of collective public interest in this area.

Developments in the Basic Scheme in Morocco

The National Fund of Social Insurance Organizations (CNOPS) manages the optional health insurance scheme for public servants in Morocco. The state as employer here pays an employer's contribution covering sickness and maternity risks. Benefits to members and those deriving entitlement from them are covered up to a maximum of 80 percent of the recognized levels for reimbursement, and even 100 percent for chronic illness.

The social security system in Morocco has to undergo a profound change as a result of developments in the economic and social sphere, especially in connection with the introduction of the compulsory health insurance scheme. The situation is critical, involving a persistent financial deficit with a direct impact on the activities of the mutual benefit societies and the CNOPS.

To cope with the changes, the roles of the main actors involved— mutual benefit societies, health care providers and the administration—must complement one another through partnerships. More importantly, the purely financial approach that has prevailed so far must not be concretized: rather, a global understanding of the problems involved in the operation of sickness insurance must be sought.

To provide its members with the best possible services, the CNOPS must continue to accommodate its obligations deriving from the principle of solidarity and adapt to a health care and protection market that is open to competition. For this purpose, it has set itself three main directions for action:

- to respond to members' new expectations and to cope with change;

- to strengthen management structures;

- to improve its image by improving the quality of its products and services.

With a systematic policy of promotion, the CNOPS hopes to be able to cope with competition and make itself better known outside its traditional spheres, for example among the different actors involved in health care. This policy will focus on the following aspects:

- the need to harmonize methods and services and to centralize the technical (computers) and financial resources covering the sickness and maternity branches;

- the need to provide safety nets to ensure financial security and to honor commitments;

- the need to improve relations with health care providers.

To attain these objectives and to play their full role in social protection, mutual benefit societies must hence have a twofold aim:

- to decentralize administration so as to improve response to members' needs, and

- to introduce efficient administration ensuring optimal use of resources and the use of computerized procedures.

As insurance techniques are becoming increasingly complex to manage, mutual benefit societies must introduce a statistically based work plan to calculate the cost of risks. In human terms, this means providing short-term training programs for administrators and considerably more long-term training for their staff.

Whether compulsory or optional, the functioning of health insurance in Morocco must be based on an obvious but essential consideration: the institution managing it must at all times have the necessary resources to meet its obligations in terms of the benefits to which its members are entitled. This means adjusting contribution levels for members and employers.

The mutual benefit scheme (governed by Dahir No. 1-57-187 of 24 Jamouda II 1383, of 12 November 1963, respecting the status of mutual benefit societies) reimburses the expenditure on health care of its members and those deriving entitlement from them. This includes primarily treatment provided by doctors and prescriptions (laboratory analyses, pharmaceuticals, treatment in health centers, etc.). The regulations require the CNOPS to reimburse 80 or 100 percent of the value where the expenditure is specified in the recognized levels for reimbursement. By contrast, the level of fees for direct consultation between doctor and patient is not set under the CNOPS scheme, and the reimbursements made for such fees hence represent only a small fraction of the full value of medical and surgical fees. For this reason, the level of such fees is below the legal level.

To halt the growth in health costs, mutual benefit societies and the CNOPS are trying to introduce a scheme, in agreement with the medical associations, based on a collective agreement as set out in section 38 of the Dahir respecting the status of mutual benefit societies. This new scheme is an opportunity for the parties involved to change their behavior, with the collective agreement (medical associations/CNOPS) replacing the direct agreements (patient/doctor). It also makes it possible to provide safety nets, as the collective agreement will place limits on excess fees.

To halt the decline in the quality of the products offered to its members, especially in view of the introduction of competition between the public and private sectors, the CNOPS has adopted a position regarding the development of its relations with health care providers, as follows:

- Policy regarding agreements between doctors and social insurance organizations has been initiated by the Ministry of Public Health, which is responsible, inter alia, for the government's social policy and the compulsory health insurance scheme project. The work of the ad hoc committee, through meetings chaired by the Minister of Public Health with all parties concerned (administration, doctors, mutual benefit societies, private-sector employer's associations), has resulted in a recommendation for the institution of a scheme based on a collective agreement.

- The CNOPS has reacted positively to the project of the Ministry of Public Health, especially as section 38 underpins this measure, which contains nothing new in itself, since relations between the CNOPS and doctors in introducing the front-end deductible payment system date back to more than four years ago when they filled the vacuum left by the CNSS in denouncing the agreement concerning treatment in polyclinics.

- The draft text of the agreement provides for the involvement of the Conseil National de l'Ordre des Médecins, and one of its main features is its conferring responsibility on doctors for the fees they receive. This policy of flat-rate payments enjoys the full support of the Ministry of Public Health and is part of its policy on controlling health care expenditure.

The collective agreement aims at:

- putting an end to the prevailing anarchic situation regarding fees;

- increasing the responsibility of doctors and of the Conseil National de l'Ordre des Médecins regarding fee rates: doctors in effect undertake to calculate their fees on the rates set in the agreement and to keep them within the amounts stipulated for specific interventions in the general list of standard medical procedures;

- rationalizing the costs of surgery, childbirth and hospitalization. Such costs are not directly linked to the application of the collective agreement, but rather to facility of access to treatment and the involvement of the private medical sector. This may relax the pressure exerted by university hospital centers and will reduce the cost of training in the public health sector.

By introducing the new fee rates, the CNOPS has ensured that doctors are not tempted to increase the costs covered by the mutual benefit societies, and it has unified the flat-rate fees. The new rates apply to all specializations, and the reimbursement criteria are established in the reference indices for each form of intervention. Efforts are being made to apply this new experiment in various sectors, including training in the public health sector, and it should benefit from greater numbers of partners joining the scheme.

Should the collective agreement approach and strategy prove inappropriate to meeting the concerns of its members, the CNOPS would be the first to reopen discussion on its contents.

In the framework of draft legislation to introduce compulsory health insurance, the CNOPS is called on to play an even greater role in monitoring the reform of sickness and maternity insurance. For this reason, it has to review its own system of administration and request the restructuring of its relations with the national administration so that it can offer its members better services and avoid being handicapped by possible competition with other providers of sickness and maternity insurance.

Hence, the CNOPS proposes to commission an operational audit with the following aims to:

- analyze its current status, and in particular its relations with the national administration, and to evaluate their impact on its management;

- conduct an operational analysis of the main functions performed to fulfil its assigned role so as to identify existing shortcomings and their main causes;

- propose internal reform measures within the CNOPS and the mutual benefit societies and in their relations in managing a common area;

- conduct a particularly detailed study of the computer systems of the CNOPS in terms of its functions, analyze any shortcomings and/or inadequacies, and propose an outline for the reform of the system and the introduction of mechanisms permitting its evolution. This outline will take into account the existing constraints, as well as the current and future needs of the fund, and will identify the new constraints that will be introduced by the project to establish compulsory sickness insurance.

The Situation in Latin America

When the term "Latin America" is used to identify the part of the American continent that includes part of North America (Mexico), Central America (except Belize) and South America (except Suriname, Guyana, and French Guyana), it is thought to confer an identity. The reality is that this large geographical area has a linguistic unity, since with the exception of Brazil it has Spanish as a common language. Leaving aside that unity, but without underestimating its importance, a wide range of features can be seen showing a real mosaic of social, economic, political and ethnic structures with genuine diversity. Even Brazil itself, with its own language, has a level of inner diversity similar to Spanish-speaking America itself.

Such considerations are useful when examining the individual aspects of the socioeconomic reality of this geographical unit, as they provide an understanding of the unequal development of certain forms of organization that reflect the different characteristics of its peoples, which in turn is a consequence of their diversity.

An analysis of the current state of development of mutual benefit systems in the region shows a tremendous variety of features and forms.

Since the sixteenth century, all the countries in the region have received large influxes of migrants, mostly from European countries bordering the Mediterranean. There was also forced migration from Africa, especially during the eighteenth century. More recently, the twentieth century has seen some migration from the Slavic countries.

These migrants joined the indigenous peoples, who themselves were at different levels of development at the time of their discovery.

Features of Mutual Benefit Societies in Latin America

The philosophical bases of mutual benefit societies were laid in Western Europe. Immigrants to Latin America from that part of the world were consequently responsible for introducing the ideas that made possible their organization and development.

Those immigrants in turn encountered different levels of socioeconomic development in the various countries of the region. One result of this is the unequal development of organizations based on the philosophy of mutual benefit that those immigrants brought with them from their countries of origin, especially in the post-Napoleonic era, when the French Revolution had sparked innovative ideas to improve the living conditions of the less fortunate.

On the basis of these European foundations, associations of persons united by their geographical, national or regional origin or by common religious or philosophical ideas were formed in the various countries of Latin America.

Thus, mutual benefit societies came into being among Italian, Spanish, Portuguese, Neapolitan, Welsh, Swiss, German, French, Catholic, Evangelical, Jewish and Masonic communities, and so on.

At first, these associations focused on the basic needs (health, housing, death allowances, unemployment benefits, etc.) faced by immigrants, most of whom had very few resources to start their lives in countries where social security simply did not exist.

The present. In 1988 a group of mutual benefit organizations from different Latin American countries took up an invitation from a number of mutual benefit societies in Argentina to attend an advisory meeting being held in Buenos Aires by an international association of Latin American mutual benefit organizations. At that meeting, the American Mutual Benefit Alliance (AMA) was formed, based in Buenos Aires.

Since the foundation of the AMA, research work has been in progress to identify existing mutual benefit organizations and to promote the creation of such organizations in the Latin American region. This has resulted in the identification of mutual benefit societies addressing various objectives, ranging from purely social aims to concrete enterprises providing health care and the construction of housing. mutual benefit societies have been found in Chile, Paraguay, Bolivia, Brazil, Costa Rica, El Salvador, Mexico and in Latin American communities in Texas (United States). Activities are also being developed to support emerging mutual benefit organizations in Paraguay and south Brazil.

Hence, it can be concluded that the old ideas of mutual benefit, brought by European immigrants in the last century and at the beginning of the present century, are alive and active to varying degrees in different countries and regions.

Health care. In the area of health care, mutual benefit societies have come into being in Argentina and Uruguay in a form that is much more active than elsewhere in the continent.

The following section will focus on the analysis of the situation in Uruguay, which merits special attention because of its health care system, which has particular features that differentiate it from the situation in other parts of the world.

Mutual Benefit Societies Providing Health Care in Uruguay

Background. Mutual benefit societies began their activities in Uruguay shortly after 1850. At first, they were established as funds to make it possible to provide help to members of the group facing any of the risks covered by the mutual benefit society (health, unemployment, death, etc.).

At the beginning of the twentieth century, the government began to pass legislation on social security, assuming responsibility for the payment of pensions, retirement benefits, unemployment insurance and allowances for births and deaths.

Gradually, the mutual benefit societies came to realize that the largest risk not covered by social security was health. Hence, the mutual benefit societies focused their benefits on the treatment of disease. For this purpose they entered into contracts with doctors and private medical centers for the services needed. They derived advantage from group contracts (lower charges) and acted like insurance companies.

As their members accounted for a considerable proportion of the population, especially in Montevideo, the capital, this created a process whereby doctors became increasingly dependent on contracts with mutual benefit institutions. This led to oligopolies of demand (the mutual benefit societies) and of supply (medical centers and group doctors).

As demand could not be regulated—people keep getting sick—the prices charged by the medical centers and doctors rose. This led the mutual benefit societies to turn their attention to other areas of activity in addition to their role as insurers, and they acquired their own medical centers. This led to hospitals that were the property of the mutual benefit societies, turning the doctors into officials of these institutions, which in turn came to own their own pharmacies and rehabilitation centers, etc.

The result was a phenomenon unique to Latin America: mutual benefit societies—not-for-profit institutions—came to own medical centers of a higher level and better quality. This meant that members of the population who did not belong to any mutual benefit association aspired to membership so as to acquire peace of mind over possible future risks and access to medical care of very high quality.

The doctors' union reacted to this situation. In 1935 a medical center was established that was the property of the doctors' union, offering a system similar to that offered by the mutual benefit societies, but with the innovation that it had the largest medical staff in the country, since any doctor who was a member of the union was recognized by the center, which like those of the mutual benefit societies was a not-for-profit institution. The difference was that the center was managed by the doctors' union instead of the mutual benefit societies.

Groups of doctors who were dissatisfied with the doctors' union medical center later began to form medical cooperatives offering services similar to those initially provided by the mutual benefit societies. Such cooperatives have expanded, especially outside the capital.

The present. Health care is currently provided by mutual benefit societies (15 percent), cooperatives and the doctors' union medical center (40 percent), the Ministry of Public Health (20 percent), military and police medical services (20 percent) and private care (5 percent).

The social welfare system managed by the Social Welfare Bank (BPS) has assumed responsibility for financing health care for private-sector workers in industry, commerce, the service sector and farming, as well as retired persons in those sectors. This is financed by contributions levied at 3 percent on workers and 5 percent on employers.

The BPS has entered into contractual arrangements for health care for these workers, both active and retired, with the mutual benefit societies and the doctors' cooperatives, as well as the doctors' union, as these institutions provide services of high quality without a profit motive.

Mutual benefit societies provide health care to only 15 percent of the population, but are a benchmark both for the quality of their services and their close attention to containing costs. Hence, the role played by mutual benefit societies is fundamental to health care in Uruguay.

By means of a per capita payment, each member is entitled to the full range of medical services, medication, surgical treatment, inpatient care, etc. There is virtually no condition that is not covered by the system.

The key role played by the institutions and their benchmark status is the major achievement of mutual benefit societies in Uruguay.

The future. The system has two major weaknesses: there is no compulsory coverage for the families of active or retired workers, nor does it provide coverage for workers in the public service.

It is to be hoped that in the coming years social security will expand in scope and extend health coverage to these groups. Opinion is already moving in this direction in some political quarters. This offers grounds for hope that the health care system will be consolidated, with the mutual benefit societies being retained as a benchmark and receiving further support alongside the doctors' cooperatives.

At the same time, a number of projects are being analyzed by the mutual benefit societies to make the institutions more efficient economically and to increase the role of prevention as a basic means of improving the quality of life.

Special attention needs to be given to the process of regional integration that is being pursued by the MERCOSUR countries (Argentina, Brazil, Paraguay and Uruguay). For the moment, such integration is taking place in the economic field and is receiving attention from various South American countries with a view to integration at a continental level. Bolivia and Chile have already joined.

The process of integration will also involve social and political integration in the not too distant future. The Uruguayan health care system may as a result be affected by integration.

As regards mutual benefit societies, the conviction is growing that associations with features deriving from the mutual benefit philosophy can provide an appropriate response to health care needs in regions where resources are scarce and not-for-profit bodies have great scope for action. This line of thought seems strengthened by the growing tendency for states to withdraw services so as to attend to the basic needs of the resident population.

As the process of integration advances and centers of decision-making move further away from communities, there is every reason to hope that the latter can organize to meet their basic needs, among which health care is of primary importance.

Community organizations of the mutual benefit type offer the enormous advantage that they can provide different solutions for each community, taking account of their specific needs and the means available.

Part 6

Transformation through Information Technology Systems

12

Possibilities Offered by New Information Technology

C. Delaveau

The end of the twentieth century is marked by the accelerating development of technologies, especially information technology. In every age power has been acquired through the possession of an asset. Information and the means of controlling it have today attained a level of strategic importance that in itself makes those who possess it capable of action and decisions.

With their origins in the market and later their generalization throughout society in the welfare state, social security and health care have long seemed removed from the problems related to this phenomenon. Yet the volume of data processed in this non-market sector accounts for three to four billion transactions each year, twice the number handled by banks. The sensitive nature of the information concerned—medical and personal data—has also served to delay the necessary evolution.

Such technologies and those who promote them today have now reached a degree of maturity allowing them to reconcile considerations of economic efficiency with the security requirements. At the same time the implications of controlling information on social security and health policy make it essential to modernize information systems. The need to take account of these aspects of the issue has led all countries to give serious attention to the introduction of new information technology.

This chapter aims to study the potential offered by a modern health information system. Structuring and using such data in a secure manner means a colossal investment, both financially and in terms of the upheavals in working methods and concerns in this sector. The potential benefits nevertheless justify the investment.

This chapter draws mainly on experience in France. The introduction of the SESAM-Vitale system in the health insurance branch is currently, in fact, the most advanced in the field of health information systems.

It will be seen that the possibilities offered by new information technology go way beyond the expected impact of the automation and externalization of routine activities in health insurance, and the result is the total transformation of health information processing systems, with implications for all those involved.

While the possibilities offered by such new information technology are promising, the prerequisites for their introduction are considerable. In addition to the material conditions necessary for the collection and storage of information there is the question of the system's administration and security. Then finally there are methodological difficulties linked to the scale of such projects, which must be addressed to derive optimum benefit from the implementation of these new technologies.

New Technologies: Exploiting the Potential

The Possibilities Offered by New Technologies Go Way beyond the Expected Impact of the Automation and Externalization of Routine Activities in Health Insurance

Major computerization projects in the field of social security generally derive from management concerns linked to increasing workload and the need to improve productivity. They have involved increasing automation of the main function, which is claims settlement—the input of data to process beneficiaries' files, including insured and retired persons, those receiving allowances and those contributing to the scheme.

After a period of reflection, a project and the allocation of resources, the introduction of new technology in the health insurance was prompted by the continuing growth of reimbursement claims on paper received each year, which since the 1980s has been growing at around 5 percent a year and totalled 1 billion in 1997. At the same time the country's economic and social situation and the decline in public finances have resulted in a scarcity of resources, while the level of demand of those insured regarding quality of service has legitimately risen.

Faced with this problem, the SESAM project (Système Electronique de Saisie de l'Assurance Maladie—Electronic Health Insurance Data System), begun in 1980, foresaw the external input of paper documents,[1] with all data being entered at source through the introduction of a computerized system (EDI) for the exchange of data with health service professionals, which was preferred to other technical solutions such as electronic document scanning systems.

The flows of claims' data handled today account for a considerable proportion of that processed by the funds—between 30 and 60 percent according to the fund. In the long term, widespread use of this type of system can be foreseen for all health care professionals, including doctors. It should also apply to most paper documents (employment accident notifications, prior notice of treatment, etc.)

The health insurance system hence began considering the modernization of its data processing facilities in the field of health care primarily as a result of legitimate and very specific aims: the need to reduce the workload entailed by internal data input by developing a system allowing for input at source and the transmission of data by computer.

This option, a management solution, was however unable to win the support of others in the health care system, especially health care professionals, who have always refused to become unpaid "auxiliaries" of the health insurance funds.

In 1993 the financial approach, which is inherent in any data processing system dedicated exclusively to managing the reimbursement of claims, showed its limitations when confronted with the new challenges facing the health insurance system. Hence, a further decisive step was taken to orient the development of the information system towards a medical approach to expenditure.

Setting aside the issue of data transmission so as to improve understanding of how to develop and use the information to best advantage has made it possible to generate interest among all those involved in the provision of health care and to secure their participation.

The Possibilities Offered by New Technologies Mean the Complete Transformation of Health Information Systems

The added value derived from the introduction of new information technologies in the field of health care lies in the large-scale and comprehensive processing of the data transmitted each day. This is essential for the global regulation of the health system based on medical control of the pattern of utilization and expenditure. The key is to learn so as to educate (and prevent), and hence be able to act.

Learning. It is essential to classify medical procedures, prescriptions and diseases by means of a standard universal coding system to identify them and interpret the evolution of situations, identify anomalies, and monitor the application of the standard medical references system (RMO).[2] This has already been done in the public hospital sector and a similar effort must now be made for ambulant care. However, this approach, which was initially introduced for the coding of prescriptions, poses problems for the coding of diseases. For the moment this can only be done by health care professionals, and is used exclusively by the medical services.[3]

This problem can be attributed to the different types of intervention: the medical service works on the basis of recognized diseases, and hence is identified by a health care professional. However, a doctor cannot always give an immediate diagnosis. Then there is the question of the accuracy of the diagnosis and the responsibility of the health care professional for errors. This objection raised by health care professionals should be seen in the context of the increasing resort to legal solutions to problems in society, health care, and relations between patients and doctors.

The creation of databases of this kind involves a number of issues.

First, in terms of public health, defining medical procedures accurately makes it possible to evaluate adherence to, and the effectiveness of, standard medical procedures and techniques used in treatment. This information in turn enables public authorities to determine policy on medications on the basis of observed facts. It also makes it possible to organize very precise nationwide monitoring of health and disease. Finally, public authorities and professionals can draw on the information necessary to adapt initial and ongoing training programs, and overall planning of health services.

Awareness of the individual practices of health care professionals and insured persons in turn enables the health insurance system to assume the role of a quality, and a vigilant and enlightened, paymaster. The measures it takes to control expenditure are based on respect for medical practice established by the scientific community.[4] Automating the control function makes requests for intervention and reports more systematic and reliable, especially in regard to the prescription and consumption of medication.

Education. New technologies make it possible not only to develop useful databases, but also to optimize their use. For this purpose all those involved now have access to the information that concerns them.

This means, first, that the patient—since a single medical file is opened belonging to each patient—knows the contents of his file and has control over them. The file, which is recorded on the smart card of every insured person, can only be modified and consulted by a health care professional entitled to do so. This feature—a complete medical record—is a precondition for quality treatment, especially in the case of serious illness involving treatment by several practitioners.[5] Improvements in coordinating treatment, especially between local medical services and hospitals, should be beneficial to the patient and also aid the financial equilibrium of the health insurance system.

Action. Finally, in addition to helping raise awareness and aid prevention, this store of information enables action. Public authorities have greater possibilities to detect and alert those concerned in the event of health incidents; health insurance institutions can draw on information to identify anomalies and untypical behavior and correct them if necessary; health care professionals have all the medical data concerning their patient and can exchange information and consult one another in making a diagnosis. On-line conferencing with several participants will especially come into its own with the implementation of a single large-scale network.

This technology also makes telemedicine foreseeable, that is, making it possible to participate remotely in diagnoses or medical interventions where no local expertise is available. This sheds new light on possible solutions to the problems involved in organizing services in the field and in medically under-equipped areas, both nationally and internationally.

The transition from computer applications for routine data processing to computerized communication systems has an impact on professional practice and on work organization for all those involved in the health care system. Indeed, it creates new relationships between them.

The Total Transformation of Health Information Systems Has Implications for All Those Involved

Health insurance. For the social security institutions, the tasks affected concern some 90 percent of the technical staff responsible for claim settlements, who themselves constitute 80 percent of their staff. The organizational consequences for processing structures are extensive.

First, the computerized data exchange systems (EDI) have been developed mainly with pharmacists, who send by computer information on prescribed medications and, in some cases, even information on the action taken by the doctor. This means that the insured person no longer has to send in a claim and can be reimbursed much more quickly.

Here it should be made clear that abolishing claim forms does not necessarily mean universal exemption from advance payment, known as third-party payment. The two are, in fact, strictly independent, and just as the third-party payment system can function without such technology, so computerized data exchange does not mean that the third-party payment system is applied everywhere. This option is dependent on strictly political considerations, which in France have always been regarded as incompatible with the founding principles of liberal medicine.

The day-to-day operations of the institutions are hence profoundly affected, and as a result focus on file management and regulating and controlling external data flow. While any estimates of productivity gains resulting from the introduction of new technologies remain a delicate issue and the subject of extensive controversy, the resulting changes are a formidable opportunity for health insurance institutions to redeploy their staff. Activities can be improved (such as client reception) and new functions will be developed for risk management and control deriving directly from the new facilities offered by information technology.

Health care professionals. Medical control of data necessarily implies some computerization of medicine. Health care professionals in particular are seeing their practices transformed profoundly by the introduction of new technologies.

In any health information system the health care professional is at the source of the information. His or her involvement and personal investment are hence of primary importance. In view of the constraints imposed by the new methods (the coding, the standard medical references system (RMO), computer transmission of claims data) the advantages conferred make the investment profitable in all senses of the term. For example, access to the social security health network and the use of specialized software can be a useful asset for diagnosis (availability of both collective and individual data concerning treatment) and prescription (counter-indications and interactions between different medications, guidance in the prescription of follow-up examinations, RMO, guide to good practices, etc.).

Moreover, the computerization of doctors' practices is an opportunity for health care professionals to modernize their accounting and administrative tools and to improve the performance of their enterprise (messaging, appointments, analysis of activities, accounting, etc.).

Patients. For patients the computerization of health care means, except in emergencies, the systematic use of their card. This is counterbalanced by the possibility of carrying on one's person a card containing all the data necessary to guarantee the best possible treatment in the event of an accident (blood group, allergies, current prescribed treatment, etc.), which obviously represents progress.[6]

The transformation of health information systems has major consequences for the behavior of all involved. Quite apart from the technical aspects concerning work organization mentioned above, the technology has an impact on the relations and balance of power between different groups in the health care system.

Initial studies show that the presence of a computer has little impact on patient/doctor relations. By contrast, although it is not yet possible to measure the effects accurately, that same computer has a radical effect on the pattern of relations between health insurance institutions and health care professionals and in general between administrators and medical staff by instituting information sharing and altering the balance of power.

New Technology: Mastering Its Use

While the possibilities offered by new technologies are promising, the prerequisites for their introduction are considerable. In addition to the material conditions necessary for the collection and storage of the information there is the question of the system's administration and security. Then finally there are methodological difficulties linked to the scale of such projects, which must be addressed to derive optimum benefit from the implementation of the new technologies.

Prerequisites for the Introduction of a Health Information System

Information gathering. A number of essential questions are raised here concerning the source of information, its reliability and its relevance.

Most of those involved in the health system have their own information system, which in many cases is incomplete or at least fragmentary, and draw up their own statistics on the basis of proprietary information. What is now involved is to make all this information available to all through a specific system of entitlement. This pooling of data brings out differences of definitions and methods of counting, etc. It becomes essential to establish common standards for coding information. An initial move is to revise the general nomenclature of medical procedures and to develop a coding system. This should bring a consensus between all concerned on the information to be made available on the network, their sources and the methods ultimately retained to verify them.

Such rigor is a precondition for any viable information system. Excessive information is difficult to understand and not very useful. It is hence essential to establish structures for the administration of the system.

At the present stage everyone is free to determine the use to which the data will be put through local and remote queries.

Computerizing people. Social security institutions and administrations are structures with existing computer equipment, which makes it possible to coordinate the migration of the equipment. By contrast, health care professionals are self-employed workers who have freedom to decide whether or not to acquire computer equipment, which they choose. This position of principle is difficult to reconcile with the introduction of health information and the constraints it implies in terms of harmonizing data and standards for its transmission.

In the absence of any move to make the contracting of health care professionals conditional on their joining the system, therefore, the question of incentives arises. The additional facilities (see below) made available are a necessary but not decisive element. The decision has been taken to provide financial assistance to health care professionals to help them acquire equipment, and to have the health insurance system pay for the transmission of electronic claims data and the associated equipment maintenance.[7]

Experience has nevertheless shown that the financial cost of computerization is only one element accounting for the reticence displayed. Misgivings among practitioners about equipment that they do not regard as an accessory for their professional practice, but rather as a tool of bureaucracy, is a key element in the refusal of some such professionals. To offset these difficulties and ensure the coherence of the data system, public authorities have made it compulsory to send claim slips by computer.[8] Nevertheless, the real answer lies in training health care professionals and in the technical assistance that the social security institutions can provide in putting the system into place.

An existing network. This is the essential material support of any information system, as it makes it possible to link those involved and to organize data collection and administration. Its efficient implementation is a technical challenge linked to the many different actors involved, their status, and the highly sensitive nature of the data processed.

There are also political aspects, since control of the data implies a leadership role.

In France two specific solutions were quickly discarded. First, the relative weakness of the Internet in France and the persistent security problems on the worldwide Web meant this option was rejected. Use of the RAMAGE network of the health insurance system was also envisaged when the project was limited to the computerized transmission of claims and the collection of data by the health insurance system. This option was also set aside when many more extensive services were included for health care professionals.

In order to place all those involved on an equal footing and in view of the development of proprietary network—including those financed by the pharmaceutical industry—the decision was made to set up a new network, the Réseau Santé Sociale (RSS—Social Security Health Network) and to assign its management to a private operator by means of a public service concession.[9]

This solution has the advantage of enjoying a consensus among all involved. However, it also presents other kinds of difficulties, including the economical and competitive pricing of a product, since access to the RSS derives from public service concerns.

System Administration and Security

Secure data flow. The creation of a unified information system based on a shared network holding sensitive data means introducing security procedures.

Several aspects must be taken into account. First, the nature of the data (individual and medical) makes it essential to monitor closely its safe transmission. For this purpose the most advanced encryption procedures must be used.[10] In addition, points of access to the network must be limited and identified.

Finally, software giving access to the network must be authorized by public authorities.[11]

Authenticating access. One absolute precondition is to define rights of access to the network for different categories of users (administrators and medical staff). However, to this must be added some device for the formal recognition of users. The most appropriate is the distribution of professional smart cards that are strictly personalized. Insured persons, doctors, researchers and administrators—everyone seeking access to the network must have the necessary means to identify themselves that grants them access to a predefined set of services. The smart card combined with a confidential code is an ideal solution, as it guarantees exclusive use by its owner, who is responsible for the transactions made under its identifying code.

It is interesting to note that, at the present stage, this technology makes it necessary to adapt legislation to avoid any risk of a legal void. In law the material basis of proof, for example the authenticity of a signature, is defined with reference to a paper medium, which is tending to become rarer.

Using the data. The methods of creating files containing data on individuals are strictly regulated and controlled.[12] The first criterion to be taken into account in designing the architecture of the databases and the related system of access entitlements is the collective or individual nature of the data. In the framework of public health policy on observing mortality rates and epidemiological phenomena, certain forms of health data are aggregated and anonymous. In this case it is possible and even desirable to provide for widespread access to such data, which are of general interest. By contrast, once the data on disease or the prescription of medication relate to individuals and names, then strict ethical rules apply not only to health care professionals, but also to the administrative staff of social security institutions.

System administration. This is a primordial function, as it consists in piloting the information system at cruising speed. In addition to constant vigilance over the quality of the data transmitted and how it is used, it also means making constant improvements in all these areas and being on the lookout for new data and potential new users. This is a strategic role, as the development of the network must not detract from its coherence or security.

The existence of a structure responsible for administering the information system is hence essential to its survival. This may prove extremely difficult to introduce on account of the many different actors involved in the health system.

This is a recurring element in the methodological difficulties encountered in managing projects of such scope.

Methodological Difficulties Encountered in Such Projects

A fragmented health system. Various types of actors are involved in the political, economic and technical spheres. The supply of health care is shared between public and private health establishments, profit-making and other. Practitioners can combine private practice with salaried employment and consultation outside the hospital. Integrating all health care professionals is made difficult by the fragmentation of their trade union representation and the lack of any agreed interlocutor.

As regards the institutions responsible for financing, these are very numerous and have widely varying status and forms of management that are specific to the professional categories for which they were founded. Compulsory basic schemes and institutions offering supplementary coverage make it a point of honor to maximize their differences when confronted with what they regard as a threat of hegemony from the general scheme.[13]

Finally, in addition to the usual compartmentalization between different administrations, the public authorities have to deal with the consequences of the deconcentration resulting from the creation of the many different agencies in the field of health care which they are responsible for supervising.[14]

The need to bring these different actors together involves more than the establishment of coordination structures. For example, the steps involved in the creation, configuration and distribution of smart cards for insured persons and health care professionals have been carried out through GIE-Sésam Vitale and GIP-CPS.

However, satisfactory in political terms, the search for a consensus and efforts to integrate all the actors involved detract from the management of these projects. Only rarely are they accompanied by a strict clarification of roles, which is essential to rapid and rational decision-making.

Control of planning. The large number of actors involved is one of the issues mainly responsible for the purely relative value of the different planning stages for such a vast project as the revision of a health information system.

Moreover, the need for a degree of maturity and coordination is in conflict with the constant evolution of equipment and of the techniques used. Evolutions in technical facilities have an impact on the balance of economic and political forces, making new decisions necessary.

In this connection, the scope of a project can make its immediate implementation difficult. Thus, a more "home-spun" project such as the simple distribution by a single scheme of a smart cardto each of its insured persons, or the general availability of computerized data exchange systems (EDI), can have a greater chance of rapid success than such an ambitious project as the transformation of a health information system.

Deployment. Finally, the method of deploying a project of such scope is also important. In addition to the aspects described above concerning the provision of assistance to health care professionals, the value of experimenting locally with networks, software and equipment has been demonstrated. Whatever constraints this involves, this method makes it possible not only to make the necessary technical adjustments, but also to gather information on the behavior and cooperation of the different actors involved.

The difficulties encountered in designing, implementing and piloting a health information system are considerable. Cultural obstacles are certainly the most formidable, since overcoming them does not depend on technical or economic solutions, but on the evolution of society itself.

Nevertheless, this transformation is in line with the course of history and cannot be interrupted. Moreover, the potential offered by the introduction of new technologies makes it justifiable to do all that is possible to ensure their integration and the social and cultural acceptance.

Notes

1. Notifications of treatment provided, invoicing notes, prior notice of treatment, etc.
2. Teulade Act of 1993.
3. Through the national software application known as MEDICIS.
4. RMOs are established by the National Agency for Health Accreditation and Evaluation (ANAES).
5. Dedicated health care networks are developing in this area, specializing in specific conditions such as diabetes.
6. Cf. Recommendation of the European Union on the generalized use of "emergency cards." In France such information will be included only with Vitale 2.
7. The health insurance system will pay health care professionals 40 centimes per standard claim transmitted, subject to a limit of FF3,000 as of 1 January 2000 (the rate as of 1 July 1999 is FF1, with a limit of FF3,750.)
8. The Ordinances of 26 April 1996 set out the principle of financial sanctions for failure to send claims by computer as of 1 January 2000.
9. The RSS contract was awarded to the Cegetel company for a period of five years.
10. The Government of France has just authorized the use of encryption methods hitherto exclusively reserved for military use.
11. In France this function is exercised by the Centre National de Dépôt et d'Agrément (National Center for Registration and Authorization), which is assigned to the Health Insurance.
12. In France the authority responsible for issuing authorizations and monitoring compliance is the Commission Nationale de l'Informatique et des Libertés (National Commission for Information Technology and Liberties).
13. This scheme for wage earners covers 80 percent of the population.
14. ARH (Agences Régionales pour l'Hospitalisation—Regional Hospitalization Agencies), ANAES (op. cit.), Agence du médicament (the Medication Agency), Agence du sang (the Blood Supply Agency), etc.

13

Building Up Telecommunications in the German Health Insurance Systems: Aims, Requirements, Barriers, Components

G. Brenner

Structure of the German Health Insurance

The German health insurance system is characterized by a large number of different structural elements and levels of decision-making. Planning and investment in hospitals is mainly the responsibility of state authorities at the land level. Physicians' offices are separate from the hospital system and independent, but bound by public-law framework legislation which is the responsibility of the federal government.

The running costs of hospitals and the services provided by physicians' practices are financed by health funds, which sign contracts at federal and land levels with hospital representatives and office-based physicians (Vertragsärzte).

These contracts include regulations governing organizational procedures and the guarantee of medical care for the population. They contain most of the provisions governing communications procedures within the health insurance system, including the regulations governing documentation—the forms needed for prescriptions, admission to hospital, referrals, prescribed treatment, etc.

There is no central regulatory authority responsible for all sectors of the German health care system. This is one of the main reasons why the introduction of telecommunications technology into the

German health insurance system is proving difficult. Owing to the large body of regulations within each sector and the differing regulatory competence of the sectors, telecommunications cannot develop freely and independently.

The Aims: Quality and Cost-Effectiveness

It is now widely believed that telematics can considerably increase the quality and cost-effectiveness of the health insurance system. By telematics, we mean a combination of information technology and telecommunications. If medical data are transmitted to the site where care is being provided, to support diagnostic or treatment procedures, it is also called telemedicine.

Quality management is becoming more important, both within a single level of care, for example, between different physicians' practices for outpatient treatment, and for the transition between levels of care, for example, between the physician's practice and the hospital. Case management is intended to achieve better control over the treatment of an individual patient, whereas disease management is intended to provide structured care for a particular diagnosis. (See Table 13.1.)

Table 13.1
Aims of the Communications Platform

Quality
- case and disease management
- guideline-based treatment
- minimum standards guaranteed
- cross-sector disease monitoring

Cost-effectiveness
- more rational organization of tasks
- no need for paper-based documentation
- reduces potential errors due to conversion between different media
- reduces duplication of work

Transparency
- morbidity analysis
- finance allocation
- needs analysis

Availability of current and past treatment data at the site of treatment is essential for quality management.

Encouraged by the Internet and a large number of very successful one-off projects, many actors in the health insurance system now want to communicate electronically, exchange treatment data and send administrative data.

Inter-Operability via Standard Interfaces

Because of the decentralized and self-managed structures which have grown up over time in the German health insurance system, there is no central, standard-setting authority that could "prescribe" the cross-sector norms and standards without which telecommunications and telemedicine are inconceivable.

These essential standards and regulations cover the following areas:

- achieving inter-operability between different systems by agreeing on uniform dataset formats and communications interfaces;

- agreeing on a security architecture which will guarantee the integrity of transmitted data, by encrypting and verifying the identity and authenticity of both sender and recipient;

- establishing and operating organizational structures for the certification of technical procedures and the accreditation of quality assurance measures. (See Tables 13.2 and 13.3.)

Nevertheless, within the various sectors of the health insurance system, the various actors have used their definition powers to create interfaces and define dataset formats which allow their associated members in the hospital or outpatient sectors a limited degree of inter-operability for the purposes of data exchange. The so-called XDT standards provide a dataset format for the exchange of administrative data and test results between practice computer systems. The National Association of Statutory Health Care Physicians and the Central Research Institute of Ambulatory Health Care in Germany have defined the ADT (invoicing data carrier) interface for the transmission of invoicing data between the office-based physician and the National Association of Statutory Health Care Physicians. The so-called BDT (standard interface for basic clinical data profiles) was developed for the transfer of test results from one practice

Table 13.2
Technical Components of the Communications Platform

Network technology
- Internet
- Intranet

Encryption software
- encryption
- digital signature

Trust center
- key management
- key distribution
- regulation of sector-specific reception centres

Standard interfaces
- format
- contents

Data cards
- identification function
- transfer function
- access authorization
- carrier function

Product certification

Table 13.3
Organizational Components for the Communications

- communication model
- application
- "standard-setting" consensus group

---

computer to another. Both these interfaces have become de facto standards in the practice computer systems currently available on the market, either because the implementation requires them or because the user has chosen them—a kind of "standardization by acceptance."

In the hospital sector, the so-called Health Level 7 (HL 7) system has become equally important. It is thus already possible to exchange substantive information to a limited extent within—but not between—the various sectors. However, these successes must not disguise the fact that the so-called XDT interfaces and HL 7 are partial solutions, confined to Germany: they are incapable of providing electronic communication over the whole country, let alone internationally.

Security Architecture Using a Certification Authority

As far as the regulatory situation allows, there is thus an urgent need to create organizational structures leading to the establishment of a single communications platform in the health care system, if communication processes are not to fall foul of these partial solutions. By "communications platform" we mean all the legal, organizational and technological components and services which enable open and—where necessary—protected and secure communication between users and applications systems in health care. (See Table 13.4.)

One has to ask oneself why no communications system of this kind has yet been set up. (See Figure 13.1.)

A crucial part of the development of the communications platform is the creation of a certification authority-that is, setting up a trust center. The trust center should be set up by all the medical and auxiliary services in the health insurance system, meeting in a consensus group and jointly determining the necessary legal, organizational and security regulations. The parties should conclude a partnership contract creating a single limited-liability certification company for the entire country, which will administer and distribute keys for all medical and auxiliary disciplines. The registration and reception center which will determine the particular characteristics of the members of each profession can then be established for each sector in accordance with agreed organizational criteria. (See Tables 13.5 and 13.6.)

Table 13.4
Communications Platform for the Health Care System

All
- legal
- organizational
- technical

Components and services for
- open
- protected
- secure

Communication between
- users
- applications systems

Figure 13.1
Communication Platform

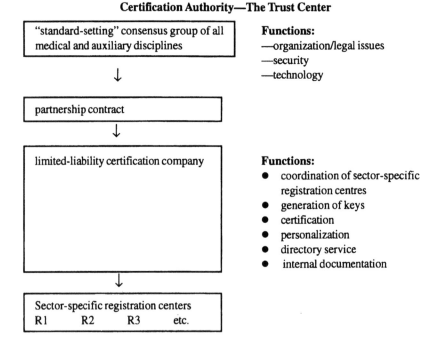

Zentralinstitut, Köln 1999

Table 13.5
Certification Authority—The Trust Center

"standard-setting" consensus group of all medical and auxiliary disciplines	**Functions:** —organization/legal issues —security —technology

↓

partnership contract

↓

limited-liability certification company	**Functions:** • coordination of sector-specific registration centres • generation of keys • certification • personalization • directory service • internal documentation

↓

Sector-specific registration centers R1   R2   R3   etc.

Table 13.6
Certificates in the Health Care System

Digital signatures
Corporations under public care
The role of physicians' corporations under public law

"Bodies which exercise control over professional activities under public law (e.g., medical associations) may operate their own certification authority to record relevant professional data in a certificate or may sign a contract of cooperation with a particular certification authority: they may encourage persons under their professional control to allow the relevant data to be recorded in a certificate by that authority only. Parties with whom these individuals wish to communicate may insist on receiving a certificate from that authority ..."

Article 3, paragraph 2, explanatory notes to the Decree on Digital Signatures

---

Promoting Telematics Projects— The First Step Towards Routine Use?

Up to now, the technology of telemedicine and telecommunications has been promoted on the assumption that successful pilot projects for digital transmission of clinical data and images between various medical providers will generate a need for this technology among the potential users. The public policy for the promotion of telecommunications assumed that the need for telecommunications would, by itself, stimulate the demand for implementation of a common communications platform for all users in the health care system who possessed the necessary basic infrastructure.

After several years of this policy of promoting telemedicine at national and European levels, we must ask ourselves why this aim has not been achieved, despite many successful pilot projects, some of which are still running. In retrospect, we can see a major error of judgment. The hypothesis that the promotion of technology and applications would, by itself, create a market for telecommunications in the health care system is a dubious one in light of the experience to date.

The technology is widely available; however, the demand among potential users (physicians, hospitals, pharmacists and patients) cannot grow by itself in the "managed market" of the health insurance system. Communication processes in the health insurance system

---

Table 13.7
Barriers to Electronic Networking

- organization of procedures governed by contracts
- sectoral responsibilities
- no standard format for medical documentation no compulsory classification systems
- no compulsory classification systems

---

are defined by conventional procedures (e.g., prescriptions written or printed on paper) which cannot be changed by the telecommunications industry or by the individual physician or pharmacist. (See Table 13.7.)

Even in areas where there is no current requirement for public-law regulation, that is, when test results are appended to a physician's referral letter, compulsory regulation by professional associations and federations or by the state would be required if new telecommunications technology were to be introduced. This would have to cover at least dataset formats, communications interfaces and encryption procedures.

Because no central political will has developed to achieve these aims, the process of agreement between the various levels of management and the various actors in the highly sectorized health insurance system is proving extremely difficult to begin. In the past, pilot projects employing high-tech telecommunications applications have actually proved to be a barrier to the necessary process of agreement.

The cases in question involved either specialist telecommunications applications which reached only a small group of users (e.g., telesurgery, teleoncology) or applications calling for structured datasets (e.g., for the treatment and monitoring of diabetic patients), which made the as yet unsolved problems of documentation in medicine glaringly obvious. It was therefore necessary to undertake a long and wearisome process of mediation between the medical experts, which did not convey to health decision-makers the imperative need for measures such as medical patient cards, with their associated infrastructure.

The reasons why these pilot telecommunications projects in medicine cannot be extended to everyday practice are due to the following factors, among others:

- Because the telecommunications applications were aimed only at specialist medical applications, the group of potential users was too small to justify the creation and financing of the necessary infrastructure on the scale which would be needed.

- The pilot projects have not, or not yet, shown that there is an economic advantage in the improved quality of patient treatment which is expected, or has been proved, to result from the availability of data in electronic form.

- The need for physicians, pharmacists and patients to participate on a completely voluntary basis, for instance in pilot projects involving patient cards, was a considerable restriction on the useful coverage of the project in the test area. If participation is voluntary, there will be problems of acceptance if any of the actors in a particular area do not join the project.

- Because the security infrastructure needed for the encryption of medical data (trust centers, certification authorities for keycards) was not available, simpler encryption procedures specific to each project were chosen, which could not provide an absolute guarantee of accuracy and authenticity of the transmitted data. This reduced acceptance because of potential liability problems.

Standardized Patient Records—An Essential Prerequisite for the Communications Platform

Up to now, telemedicine has been seen as a collection of one-off, isolated applications making use of information and communications technology. This view has unfortunately disguised the true potential of telematics which, viewed as a whole, can offer a way of solving current major problems in the health care system, such as lack of transparency, integration and control.

Telematics can improve the quality and coverage of medical care and, at the same time, make care more cost-effective by making all relevant patient information available at the site of treatment. This will require communication and cooperation, as well as the introduction of integrated electronic patient records and a management system which will allow authorized users access to these records.

Guidelines, compilations of information and knowledge-based systems can provide information for medical care which is relevant to individual cases. Supplementing anonymous information derived from the patient records of all insured persons with system-description data will allow planning and decision-making in the health care system to be based on disease-related data. The successful use of telecommunications to optimize this potential will require the creation of a communications platform centered on integrated multi-media electronic patient records.

Multimedia electronic patient records allow all data relating to the patient's health, which are currently distributed among different media in different places, to be logically combined. In the electronic patient record, all information about a patient is documented in digital form, following an identical dataset format. The various items of information can be linked to one another by means of an identification key and assigned to individual patients. Electronic patient records may be, but do not have to be, archived in a single place. All data relating to patients and information relevant for insurance benefits are documented in the patient record, which is usually stored in a decentralized fashion by the various service providers. The collected data and information can be called up with reference to a particular individual or anonymously. This provides an important foundation not only for medical treatment, but also for administrative matters relating to services and invoicing in health care.

In the first stage of the project, all information available in digital form is added to the computerized patient record. In the second stage, information which cannot be made available in digital form is stored as images in a data-processing system, which can be called up from various places. The introduction of electronic patient records brings a number of requirements and problems to be solved, including the following. (See Table 13.8.)

Data cards are an essential part of the communications platform, as are identification cards or patient keycards. The patient keycard is a physical expression of ownership. The patient holding the card (pointer card) possesses the key to any information directly related to himself/herself, stored in a number of different places.

Table 13.8
Multimedia Patient Records—A Prerequisite for Network Communication

- documentation of patient data and test results with standard formats, structures and classification in all health facilities
- a single identification system for patients
- guarantee of data integrity
- regulation of access and update authorization
- access control by means of the physician and patient identification cards

The Way Forward to the Communications Platform—A Simple Application

Although it has not proved possible to extend the private and public pilot projects into everyday practice, they have contributed a great deal, not only to the accumulation of the necessary technical experience, but also to the realization that, if telecommunications are really to be used in the German health insurance system, it is absolutely essential to promote the organizational infrastructure needed for a communications platform common to all actors in all sectors of the health insurance system.

This aspect should receive particular attention in research and promotion policy in the future. We therefore make the following recommendations:

- The aim of introducing telemedicine and telecommunications into the German health care system and ensuring their widespread use must be kept firmly in mind.

- Projects which will lay the foundations for a common communications platform—a basic infrastructure serving a large number of users—should be promoted.

- These foundation elements include:

  — Definition of encryption procedures

  — Establishment of trust centers and certification authorities to issue and administer keycards for all actors who send or receive medical data

  — Implementation of standard and universal communications interfaces for the exchange of medical data

  — Definition of the dataset structure

- A comparatively simple medical application could be selected as a "shoehorn" solution to achieve the aim of building up a communications platform, while avoiding the as yet unsolved problems of documentation and classification of diseases. A simple application should fulfil the following criteria. (See Table 13.9)

Table 13.9
Criteria for Applications Which Would Pave the Way for
the Communications Platform

- Involve a number of sectors in the health system
- Involve patients
- Choose a set of data which need to be transmitted several times a day
- Simple and standardized dataset structure
- Existing, generally accepted classification system
- Provable economic advantage
- Qualitative benefit
- Requirement for all the technical elements of communication

---

The Electronic Prescription—The First Step Towards a High-Coverage Communications Platform

The "shoehorn" function described above could be fulfilled by an electronic prescription. However, it is important that this shoehorn application, which is intended merely to set up a common infrastructure, should not be seen as a solution in its own right. For this reason, the communications platform should not be designed so that it allows the electronic prescription application and no other. The actors in the health care system must first define an overall strategy covering all the likely applications.

An infrastructure following this design would create a communications platform which would allow telecommunications to be used for special applications and small numbers of users, or allow electronic letters to be exchanged between physicians, as soon as the dataset format needed for this has been agreed. When the electronic prescription is introduced, all the components of the telecommunications system (Intranet, encryption, trust centers, certification authority, communications server, universal communications interfaces, hardware and software) must be made available to physicians' practices, pharmacies and hospitals. Existing elements can be incorporated into the system, such as the German Health Network as the Intranet, standard communications interfaces such as BDT, existing pharmaceutical information systems as a classified pharmaceutical database or existing computer centers as communications servers.

Scenarios for the Electronic Prescription

The organizational design for the development and introduction of an electronic prescription is intended to replace the existing paper-based prescription and invoicing system. Using a rough estimate of the amount of work involved in the current system, one can expect modern, integrated data processing and data transfer methods to achieve savings of approximately one-third of current costs. Two models are under discussion:

- an online prescription communication service connecting the physician's practice, the pharmacy, the insurer and the Association of Sickness Fund Physicians by means of a central server or a number of connected decentralized computers (server model)

- communication of prescriptions between the physician's practice and the pharmacy using a chipcard (card model).

Server model (see Figure 13.2)

The physician decides which drugs to prescribe. By means of the Health Professional Card, he/she is identified to the system as a physician, generates an electronic prescription and signs it using a digital signature. The patient's insurance card is read into a card reader at the physician's practice. Together with the physician's Health Professional Card, it gives the physician's practice computer access to a "prescription server." The physician enters the prescriptions into the database on this server. When the patient goes to a pharmacy and is identified by means of the patient card, the pharmacist is likewise identified by means of a Health Professional keycard and, using the patient card, can gain access to the prescription server and the database containing the patient's information, thus finding the prescription and dispensing the drugs. The prescription is then marked as dispensed, which prevents the patient going to another pharmacy and asking another pharmacist to dispense the same drugs again.

The pharmacist saves the prescription in an internal pharmacy file and uses it, along with other necessary information, to invoice by the sickness insurance fund in respect of drug costs.

Card model (See Figure 13.3)

When the physician has decided which drugs to prescribe and has been authorized by means of his/her Health Professional Card,

Figure 13.2
Electronic Prescription—Server Model

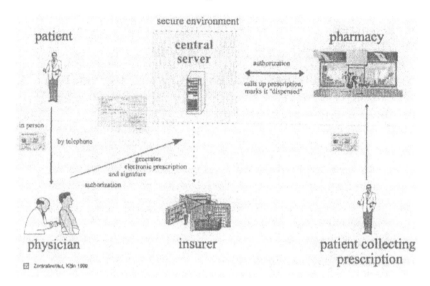

Figure 13.3
Electronic Prescription-Card Model

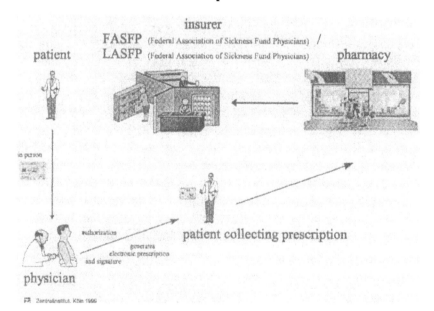

he/she enters an electronic prescription on the patient's pharmacy card, verifying it with a digital signature. The patient can obtain the drugs from a pharmacy by producing his/her pharmacy card. The pharmacy's invoice to the insurer is processed in the same way as at present, through the pharmacy computer centers.

The card model has the advantage over the server model that it does not require the operation of a server system, with the accompanying organizational work. However, the card model makes less of a contribution to rationalization, since although the prescription data are issued, stored and read electronically, central data holding and central data access to anonymous data for the purposes of invoicing and monitoring (e.g., for budgetary control) are only possible over a second network installed in parallel. The security architecture (Healthcare Professional Cards, digital signatures and the establishment of certification authorities to manage the keys) is the same in both models.

The sickness insurance card cannot be used in the card model, since it is not permitted to store prescription information there. Consequently, either the law would have to be changed to allow the sickness insurance card to be used, or a pharmacy card would have to be introduced on a voluntary basis. Experience with such voluntary cards has shown that one cannot expect all insured persons to use the card, so it would be necessary to introduce the card model alongside the existing system, thus nullifying any economic advantage.

The card model would be suitable only for electronic prescriptions, whereas the server model would be the first step on the way to a full communications platform.

Even if the server model is the ultimate goal, it can probably only be achieved by means of the card model, since testing of any model will require a consensus about that model among the various actors (Federal Association of Sickness Fund Physicians, Association of Professional Representatives of German Pharmacists, Statutory Sickness Insurance Fund). Approaching the electronic prescription by way of the card model is also beneficial because it provides important elements of the communications platform (e.g., encryption procedures, physician identification, trust centers). If prescription data can be transferred from the physician's computer to a chipcard and read off the card back into the computer, this means that the standardized preconditions for communication have been fulfilled, and it would be possible to transfer the prescription data online between two computers or over an Intranet. Replacing the physical transfer of prescription data on to the chipcard with an online transfer to a server would be a later stage in the optimization of the communications platform. This step-by-step approach to achieving the ultimate aim would also have the advantage that the introduction of electronic prescriptions and the construction of the communications platform would not be jeopardized by conflicts of interest arising from the legal and organizational problems associated with access authorization, data protection and secondary use of the centrally stored prescription data in the server model.

A pilot project is needed so that the system can subsequently be made compulsory, as the sickness insurance card is, and introduced in the various regions at different times, in the interests of logistical organization. It must be compulsory—whether its compulsory nature is derived from a central contract between associations at the highest level or from statutory regulation—because this is the only way that a "market" can arise, with its associated synergistic effects on all the participants: industry, investors/service providers, regulatory bodies and data protection authorities.

Initiatives in Electronic Communication

In the Federal Republic of Germany today, a large number of different initiatives can be identified for the creation of an electronic communications structure in the health care system.

More than 80 percent of physicians' practices and hospitals are now equipped with data-processing technology, which means that the majority of medical facilities now have the basic equipment needed for electronic data holding, processing and management. The use of Internet technology is increasing. Supplementing the use of the Internet, intranets specific to a particular profession or field (e.g., the German Health Network) are being built up. The reason why intranets are being used is the high degree of security required for the transmission of diagnoses and test results.

For many years, invoicing and prescription data have been processed on a very large scale by computer centers for physicians, pharmacists and hospitals, and are exchanged for the purposes of invoicing the sickness insurance funds. Data transfer from the service provider to the computer center is still often paper-based, but most are now on diskette, and in a few cases data are transferred online.

The patient and his/her personal data are identified by reading in a memory chipcard on the so-called sickness insurance card. This card was introduced throughout the country in 1994/95.

Efforts are currently under way to establish a cross-sector consensus and decision-making group, consisting of representatives of associations of sickness insurance funds, physicians, hospitals and pharmacists, in order to reach a consensus about the central norms and standards which are required and introduce them in the various sectors on a self-regulatory basis. The most basic requirements for a security architecture—the creation and equipping of certification authorities (trust centers) to administer private and public keys for all members of the medical professions, as well as electronic signatures and encryption of patient data, are being defined. An initial version of the specification for the Health Professional Card, developed for German physicians by the Society for Mathematics and Data Processing, is now available.

An important milestone in the establishment and operation of certification authorities in Germany was the adoption of the Law on Digital Signatures in 1997. This law specifies the requirements which must be fulfilled in order to operate a certification authority, the key management procedure and the validity of the electronic signature.

Parallel with the development of components of the future electronic communications platform, publicly promoted reports have given rise to widespread public debate about the applications of telematics in the health care system. Here we should mention a report on telematics applications in the health care system produced by the management consultants Roland Berger & Partners on behalf of the Federal Ministry for Health and the Federal Ministry for Research and Technology, and the INFO 2000 discussion group set up by the federal government.

A research initiative by the Federal Ministry for Research and Technology on the creation of medical communications networks for a number of clinical applications is intended to clear the way for an electronic communications platform from the scientific side and install the necessary components.

In the end, the spread of electronic communication in the health care system will depend on finding answers to the following crucial questions.

- Who will verify the identity of participants, and using what methods?

- How can secure network communications be guaranteed?

- How can patient data and test results be exported and imported between different applications systems?

- Can a single certification authority be set up for all users?

- What is the evidential value of electronically transmitted clinical data?

14

Data Protection and Data Security in Shared Care Information Systems

B. Blobel

Changes in the Structures and Function of the Health Care and Social Welfare Services and in the Architecture of Their Information Systems

Health care and social welfare services in all parts of the world-to different degrees and each with their own set of problems—all face growing challenges and changing, usually more stringent, structural conditions. The underlying causes of these more stringent circumstances and increased demands are manifold, and range from changes in the socioeconomic structure (culture, generation relationships, age structure) and increasingly more demanding ways of viewing progress in medicine and medical technology to population explosions accompanied by comparative impoverishment of large sections of the population and the need to guarantee primary care and satisfy the corresponding need to make up the differences. The answer to the challenges-at least in the developed and newly industrializing countries-is the same: raise quality and efficiency in the health care processes and aim to diminish costs by

- differentiating the protection structures (social laws, architecture of social security);

- specialization and decentralization of the health care services, together with

- integration of the health care services through increased

- communication and cooperation within and between the institutions of the health and social welfare services.

The Shared Care Paradigm

The health insurance and social welfare system described above, which is based on the division of labor and inter-linked establishments, is realized in the Shared Care Paradigm (Blobel 96 a, b, e; Blobel 97 a). Shared care, according to (Ellsässer 93), is the "continuous and coordinated activity of different people in different establishments using different methods at different times in order to be able to provide the best possible medical, psychological and social assistance to patients."

This development requires and furthers at the same time:

- development and application of medical, technical and administrative (quality) standards on which to base

- transparency of process and performance in order to establish and realize the requisite professional relationships, and

- active controlling of the highly dynamic structures and processes that may arise.

There are also various trends towards free market principles and competition, which we do not, however, intend to deal with in this chapter.

The system architecture of a particular health care and social welfare system defines the structural conditions. In health care system architectures that are largely centralized through contracts and funding, as for example in Great Britain within the framework of the National Health Service initiatives (with slight variations from one region to another), there are clear structures as well as standard functional schemes. The needs of the health service and the requisite structures are worked by Regional Health Authorities. The interaction between the various medical services is managed by a registered doctor who is contracted to each individual patient in the same way as the ("Hausarzt") general practitioner in Germany. In the highly fragmented and at the same time federally organized German health insurance and social welfare system, which has a private primary care sector, a secondary care area with complex organizations and legal systems, and equally diverse care services, managing the link-up into a shared care system turns out to be an exceptionally difficult matter.

This finds expression, amongst other places, in the protracted and complicated discussions on the corresponding initiatives and draft laws. Both the state and the organization concerned have a decisive role to play in defining the structural conditions (needs and structural planning, health care commitment). The ways in which interactions operate are established by negotiation and the agreements arising from them between the service areas and between the latter and the cost units or other relevant establishments under the controlling influence of the respective interested parties.

At the present time the German federal government supports the key function of the general practitioner as patient advisor and navigator in the currently emerging Shared Care model of using groups to optimize practical patient care. In order to fulfil this function the navigator requires comprehensive information about the patient, that is, access to the complete electronic health record of the patient. As this data base is highly sensitive and may also contain social data, for example relating to drug abuse or similar issues, only the patient and the responsible doctor (preferably the general practitioner) should have access to this information, for the ethical and legal reasons set out below (Blobel 96 a; Blobel 99 a, c).

In Germany the Managed Care model is being tested as a special form of care pathway and practical management of the shared care system, where the insurance companies as cost units could take on the role of actively advising and guiding the patient. But just for these very reasons there are strong reservations on the subject.

The rather static shared care architecture of American managed care, which is based on the contractual (and therefore limited) established structure of a health maintenance organization (HMO), should not be taken as much more than a point of reference.

Sweden is currently developing regional structures for the organization of an inter-linked health care system to treat patients under shared care.

Shared Care Health Information Systems

The required health care information systems must meet political and administrative needs and must therefore also be communicative and interoperable. The current trend is therefore to separate interoperable health information systems and health care networks. The system architecture of a particular country's health and social welfare system defines the architecture and function of the communication and cooperation infrastructure. Thus, in a largely cenralized environment, the British health service has, or is developing, a communication network with specific interfaces, protocols and communication content.

The German health insurance system, on the other hand, with its separate services and democratic federally organized structure, limits the creation of link-ups, at least in the first instance, to comparable establishments (groups of hospitals under the same funding, doctor's surgery networks, etc.) where communication and cooperation are controlled on a legal basis by contracts or statutes. In this system interoperability is built up step by step, starting with simple computer-based consultation, cooperative diagnosis and therapy and going all the way up to comprehensive (unified) electronic patient records. Even the establishments involved do not in themselves constitute a formal information unit. Communication and cooperation arise out of the practical requirements of caring for a shared patient. Communication with partners outside the group has to take place in accordance with specific compulsory regulations.

Within the aforementioned architecture of a health maintenance organization in the United States a shared care group forms an information unit within which personal medical data may be freely communicated while protecting individual rights.

In shared care information systems, the concepts of data security and data protection that arise out of legal and ethical requirements and political, social, organizational and technical circumstances, and also out of the need for trustworthiness when sharing information, must be guaranteed to a high degree (Barber 96; Blobel 95 a, b; McCurley 95). Because of developments in political and economic integration these issues of secure communication and cooperation within distributed health care information systems need to be considered not only in a national but also in an international (or at least European) context.

The aspects of data security for health information that need to be guaranteed are:

- integrity of information;

- confidentiality of information;

- availability of information, and

- responsibility for information and processes in the sense of reliability and accountability.

Confidentiality of information raises certain data protection issues. Integrity and availability of information have become major criteria in health care. This is especially true where we have increasing integration of data processing into normal working procedures and a resulting dependency on correctly processed information at the right time and at the right place. So we should not limit our attentions to the extent of data protection, but integrate the question of data security into the bases for cooperation.

Basic Legal Principles for the Processing of Personal Medical Information

In the Federal Republic of Germany, as in many other countries (e.g., [CoA 88, USC 74]), freedom of the individual is guaranteed by specific privacy laws. In this the federal and local data protection laws actually go back a long way and serve as a model on an international scale. Information aspects of Article 1 of the Constitution (Human Dignity and Human Rights) and Article 2 (Rights of the Individual) are covered by these data protection laws. In addition the Federal Constitutional Court, on the basis of a referendum, has defined the civil right of the individual to self-determine information. These notions have been taken up by the European Union and, together with advanced data protection laws in many instances using the German data protection laws as a model, have been formulated into a legally binding EU directive (Barber 96; Blobel 95 a; CE 95) protecting the individual during processing and exchange of his personal data. According to this directive personal data may only be collected for a clearly defined statutory purpose, and may not be processed for any reason other than that purpose. The general ban on collecting and processing sensitive data can only be lifted if

- the patient or his representative is fully informed and has given his voluntary written consent in a form that can be verified;

- data collection or processing for medical or health-related purposes is done by persons who are bound by professional secrecy (e.g., the Hippocratic oath) or by a similar obligation;

- protection of the patient's vital interests makes data collection and data processing necessary;

- there is an inalienable statutory common interest above the interests of the individual, or there are other exceptional legal circumstances that require this data collection and processing.

At the same time data collection and data processing must be handled in a fair and just way and should be purpose-related, appropriate, relevant and restricted to the minimum. The data must be exact and may only be stored for a particular purpose and for an absolutely essential period of time. They should preferably be collected from the data subject in person and not from third parties (SGB X, §67a).

Patient Rights

The patient has the right to be informed about the intention to collect and process his personal data and also to have his rights taken into account regarding the purpose of data collection and data processing. The patient may have direct access to the data or access them via a trustworthy person such as his general practitioner. He is entitled to correct information and where necessary to remove it. As a result of the increasing penetration of information technology into medical processes, patient data may become increasingly free-standing so that the data take on a status personae and should be endowed with the rights of the individual. For this reason the EU directive says that a computer-based result that uses stored data alone is inadmissible.

The patient is entitled to expect his personal health care data to be handled with the greatest circumspection and confidentiality. The patient can also require the existing necessary information to be available at the right time and place and in the right form for the authorized person, in order to ensure the best possible treatment. Equally the personal data of those involved in the health care process must be protected according to the data protection laws.

Obligations of Health Care Workers

In order to be able to fulfil its obligations a departmentally organized health care service requires relevant information on the patient, specific parts of his case history and diagnostic and treatment information contained in the treatment record. The Hippocratic oath (§203 Abs.1 No. 1 StGB[1]) and data secrecy laws (§5 BDSG[2]) only allow health care staff to process patient data within the stated purpose of the treatment plan. Any unrestricted exchange and use of patient data, that is to say exceeding the immediate purpose, is prohibited. For this reason a hospital or even more so a shared care group cannot be considered an information unit. Here the differences between this and other structural models, such as the American one, become obvious.

The debate on data protection is made even more complicated by the tricky allocation of roles in medical information processes. Role allocation relates to varying distances from the information source; rights and duties are defined and compulsory rights to information (still regarded in Germany as property rights) have to be justified (Bakker 95). These distances must be particularly taken into account when data are used by other establishments, such as the health insurance schemes, that are indirectly involved in the care plan. For this reason medical communication and cooperation between hospitals and insurance schemes in Germany is moderated by the insurance companies' medical service.

A special area is emergency medicine, where the doctor-patient relationship is in the first instance anonymous, a fact that must be taken into consideration in concepts of security.

The patient as the original source and the health care staff as the generators of information carry the responsibility for the correct use of data and respect for the individual rights of the persons involved. It follows that only the doctor who generates the data, that is to say who collects it, or the establishment or the patient himself can authorize access to the patient's medical data and define its use. This applies also to archived data (Bakker 95; Barber 96).

In the Federal Republic of Germany communication between the service providers and the cost units also needs to be regulated within the context of the existing constitutional data protection laws. The rule is for social secrecy (social data secrecy), with communication restricted exclusively to authorized persons in accordance with the "need to know" principle, that is, minimizing the information. Cost units, such as for example the health insurance schemes, are bound to observe the compulsory regulations. For the required communication to take place they need the relevant legislation; in other words at each request for information they must quote the appropriate article and paragraph under which the information may be issued. Where an item of information is freely requested there must be explicit mention of this. In spite of this comprehensive and in some ways exemplary law there are complaints at all levels that in the course of the developments initially described the principle of subsidiarity inherent in the data protection laws undermines and diminishes the rights of the individual by applying other legal principles (BfD 95; LDSH 99).

Compulsory Basis for Social Data Communication in Germany

In the Federal Republic of Germany the laws for social data protection are generally formulated in the general section of the Social Code in Volume I Sozialgesetzbuch-Allgemeiner Teil (SGB I), §§ 35 and 37 and also in Volume X Sozialgesetzbuch Zehntes Buch (SGB X), §§ 20, 21, 67-85a. Specific protocols for personal data protection serve as the new legal basis for the additional principles mentioned above. They sometimes seem dubious and if too widely interpreted may be open to criticism.

These protocols concern compulsory health insurance (Social Code-Volume V (SGB V), §§ 73, 106, 276, 277, 284-305), the compulsory pension scheme (Social Code-Volume VI (SGB VI), §§ 147-152), child and youth welfare (Social Code-Volume VIII (SGB VIII), §§ 61-68), community care insurance (Social Code-Volume XI (SGB XI), §§ 93-109), social assistance (Federal Social Welfare Law—Bundessozialhilfegesetz, §§ 116, 117) and the compulsory application of these laws (Gesetz zur Ausführung des Bundes-sozialhilfegesetzes, §§ 2, 3a), and also the associated legislation for computerized reconciliation of data (e.g., the data reconciliation application order—Datenabgleichsdurchführungsverordnung and the social welfare data reconciliation order—Sozialhilfedatenabgleichsverordnung). All these laws and regulations, in particular SGB I, SGB V and SGB XI are relevant to the subject matter of this chapter.

Communication within the Health Care System:
Risks, Threats, and Protected Items

Communication within the health care system varies depending on the content of the communication, the partners involved, the infrastructure used and the services called upon. The contents of communications may refer to medical matters in general or to particular individuals, depending on the presence of personal data, and in particular differentiate by identification data, administrative data, social data, medical data or genetic data. With regard to the content of communications one can distinguish

- patient-related medical communications (e.g., information on diagnosis and treatment);

- patient-related non-medical communications (e.g., invoices to patients);

- non-patient-related medical communications (e.g., epidemiological results) and;

- non-medical communications (e.g., orders for materials and equipment).

In all these communications the level of sensitivity corresponding to particular protection needs must be defined from the point of view of the patient, the health care worker or the organization. Generally speaking the military classification is used: public information, confidential (internal) information, secret information and top secret (classified) information. From the patient's point of view (social data protection) the scale of sensitivity follows the above pattern.

Communication partners can be located within the health care services (e.g., doctors, hospitals, insurance schemes) or outside the health care services (e.g., suppliers, libraries). In detail communication may be distinguished according to communication between partners

- within a medical department;

- in various medical departments of a health care establishment (e.g., doctors' communications);

- in various medical and non-medical departments of a health care establishment (e.g., communication between a medical department and the accounting department);

- in various health care establishments directly involved in patient care (shared care);

- in various establishments in the health care system providing direct or indirect medical care (e.g., communication between pharmacists, laboratories etc.);

- in various medical and non-medical establishments in the health care system (e.g., communications with cost units (health insurance schemes, the Ministry of Health), or

- in various health establishments and institutions outside the health care services (e.g., suppliers, libraries)

depending on the various legal bases with various restrictions with regard to the content communicated and the right to communicate. The right to communicate sensitive, in this case personal medical information decreases down the given scale.

The communication infrastructure relates to the system architecture and the communication connections used, where the services of electronic mail may range from message systems such as HL7,[3] xDT[4] or XML[5] to shared cooperative systems based on CORBA,[6] DCOM, ActiveX components[7] or DHE[8] (Blobel 96 c, d), or possible combinations. Details of the communication infrastructure and the common communication services that are of lesser interest within the context of this chapter are given in (Blobel 97 b).

The various communication contents, partners, infrastructure elements and services may be combined in any way desired and lead to different threats and different risks, which therefore require different countermeasures.

When communicating between health care delivery systems and the health insurance schemes using the given systems there are already important restrictions that need to be placed on communication content and communication rights. This relationship, which reflects the European cultural view, is in clear contrast to the Managed Care model. More recent American legislation and standardization in health care aims at improvements which in general are nonetheless behind notions in Europe (ASTM E 1869, ASTM PS 101, ASTM PS 108, USC96).

Domain Models for Health Information Systems

In order to be able to control the architecture of communicating and cooperating medical information systems it is useful to group organizational or technical units into domains using common criteria and to operate within this framework. From the point of view of data protection and data security it is possible to define policy domains (domains with the same or an agreed policy), environment domains (domains with the same environment conditions) and technology domains (domains with the same technology). The policy, which in heterogeneous architectures is the decisive group feature, specifies the legal, ethical, social, administrative, functional and technological conditions for trustworthy communication and cooperation (Blobel 97 b, Blobel 99 b).

Domains can be grouped into super-domains, where by policy bridging a new policy has to be defined with as a rule more restricted rights and extended obligations. It is also possible to define sub-domains. A domain is interpreted as having defined conditions (threats and risks) and as thereby being controllable, so that protective measures are only necessary at the borders with connections to the outside environment. A typical example of this view are the so-called virtual private networks (VPN, Intranets), which are protected by fire walls against the policy-free Internet.

The trend in information systems is however towards architectures with end-to-end security, so that no further assumptions need to be made regarding the network environment and the Internet with its fast-evolving opportunities can be used (Blobel 98 b; Katsikas 98). In this context it is also very revealing that more than 70 percent of the attacks on health information systems are perpetrated by insiders (cf. the sections below).

Threats and Risks in Health Information Systems

Amongst the threats to data protection and data security in health care one can distinguish between actions that occur by chance, on the spot, with little criminal motivation (negligence) and aggressive directed attacks with a high criminal motivation (intent). Threats of the first type arise through

- unauthorized outsiders to the establishment (e.g., chance visitors at unsupervised equipment or a client getting a view of a screen that shows other cases, e.g., if reception places in a hospital or customer advice slots in a health insurance office are thoughtlessly entered);

- unauthorized members of staff (e.g., non-medical personnel and personnel without special authorization);

- members of staff authorized to a different area (e.g., systems managers, administrators);

- non-members of staff authorized to a different area (e.g., service personnel, maintenance personnel).

Threats of the second kind are also real and must be taken into consideration, but according to the results of international research (published as so-called incident reports) they are of a lesser nature as regards frequency (<20 percent) and also to some extent their effects. Distinguishing the types of threats is of secondary importance anyway, as the data protection laws in principle demand the best possible state of the art security.

Amongst negligence threats to data protection and IT security posed by authorized persons user errors rate very high, affecting integrity of the data and systems. There is also insufficient transparency for the user in the behavior of in-house systems and applications in use within the establishment (for example remains of text passages that have been deleted during word processing and are no longer recognizable) and the unintentional side effects of user actions (e.g., overwriting an existing data file with the same name when transferring data).

Intentional threats include deliberate manipulations by insiders who for example want to conceal their responsibility for mistakes they have made and also frustration reactions by employees. Outside threats to confidentiality, integrity and availability of data and systems occur mainly at connections to open networks. CERT advisors (CERT) have recently issued repeated warnings to be constantly on the look-out for net activities that automatically test computers linked to the Internet for security gaps.

Risks refer to the specific evaluation of threats that are realized, that is events that have occurred through the person affected, such as a user and/or an organization. The risks that information technology may bring to the health care system are above all:

- harm to a patient through faulty procedures or incorrect or incomplete data;
- the difficulty of tracing responsibility for measures taken;
- the threat to confidentiality, in particular the breach of professional secrecy and infringement of data protection laws, and
- non-availability of data or of the information system.

The results for the establishments concerned may include:

- image loss;
- financial loss from liability claims or through image-related loss of contract and therefore loss of income;

- interruptions to work procedures, with intellectual and material consequences;

- and others (SEISMED 96).

Under items to include in data protection the most important are patient data, but also data relating to personnel within the establishment, which are protected from unauthorized viewing by the data protection laws. Also under protection are the administrative and financial data of the establishment and all data processing equipment in use. In every instance of access management of systems, functions and data must be governed by the need-to-know principle or the principle of minimum rights: a data item can strictly only be viewed or changed by the person whose explicit job it is to do so (Blobel 95 a; Pommerening 91;Seelos 91). In this context the number of people who have access to personal medical data must be kept to a minimum. This can be done, for example, by assigning named insurance scheme personnel to particular patients. This kind of measure can also add to quality.

Data that derive from user activity records are also subject to data protection laws. They may be used only where it can be justified to prove breaches of security, but not to set up activity and movement profiles of workers (cf. Industrial Constitutional Law— Betriebsverfassungsgesetz). In order to settle these problems it is sometimes necessary when introducing new information systems to draw up in-house agreements between workers' representatives and management.

Information Flow in Compulsory Health Insurance

Data flows in compulsory health insurance can take many forms and in the realization of the shared care paradigm are becoming more comprehensive and above all more intensive. In the area of communication and cooperation with those medical partners directly involved in the care process, this results in the implementation of a patient-oriented, distributed, interoperable multimedia patient records, which can be accessed within the context of a developed security policy with restricted rights.

Figure 14.1 shows data flows in the area of compulsory health insurance in the Federal Republic of Germany. It should be noted here that in the German health insurance system there is an area of private health insurance, although this is relatively small. Both areas

Figure 14.1

Data flow in compulsory health insurance in the Federal Republic of Germany, adapted according to (BfD 95), with KV* = German Compulsory Health Care Administration, KZV** = German Compulsory Dental Health Care Administration, and DPC*** = Data Processing Centre.

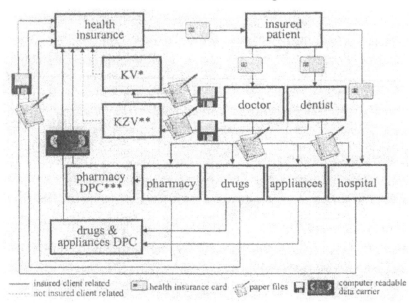

have certain features in common, although the private system is governed by the principle of reimbursement of expenses. In this chapter the discussion is limited to compulsory health insurance.

At present there is a mixture of paper-based and electronic communication of the required information, which, however, is increasingly going over in a more distant future into a completely computerized system of communication.

The data flows must have a legal basis, which may range from the treatment plan between the patient and the medical service providers or separate declarations of consent to specific compulsory regulations and administrative guidelines. The compulsory bases for communication with the compulsory health insurance schemes in the Federal Republic of Germany are given for pharmacies in SGB V, § 300, for suppliers of drugs and appliances and other service providers in SGB V, §302, for hospitals, disease prevention and rehabilitation clinics in SGB V, § 301 and for doctors and dentists in SGB V, § 295.

In the context of the compulsory regulations, the relevant organizations or their interested groups had to work out concrete application guidelines at national level in conjunction with the various structures at local government level (e.g., the Association of Compulsory Health Insurance Schemes—Dachverband der Gesetzlichen Krankenkassen, the German Hospital Corporation—Deutsche Krankenhausgesellschaft DKG, or the German Compulsory Dental Health Care Administration—Kassenzahnärztliche Bundesvereinigung KZBV). These guidelines are intended to cover in detail all aspects of data protection and data security.

For communication between hospitals and health insurance schemes the relevant interested groups of the German Hospital Corporation and the Union of Compulsory Health Insurance Schemes worked out message definitions and data exchange formats along the lines of EDIFACT, which specify content and interaction as defined in SGB V, §301. In order to manage the information flow between the various hospitals and the different compulsory health insurance schemes, including private health insurance, a clearing center was established that does not have interpretation access to the encrypted data but merely carries out the data reconciliation, grouping and routing (Figure 14.2). The architecture described here has

Figure 14. 2.
Workflow of Electronic Data Exchange within the German Health Insurance System (SGB V § 301)

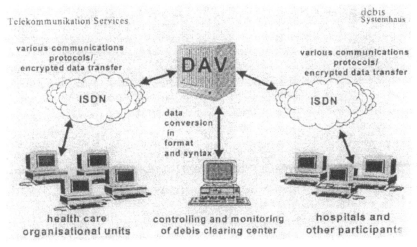

Source: debis Systemhaus.

been successfully tested in a model set up using debis Systemhaus as a clearing center. A generally applicable implementation, satisfying the above compulsory regulations, has yet to be achieved.

The organization shown in Figure 14.2 of services, materials and payment flow means that communication between the compulsory medical and dental practitioners' organizations is related to the episode of medical care, not to the patient. When SGB V, § 301 is applied the insurance information on the patient's case history derived from data processed in the Compulsory Health Care Administration (Kassenärztliche Vereinigung KV) or Compulsory Dental Health Care Administration (Kassenzahnärztliche Vereinigung KZV) is no longer anonymous. However, the KV and KZV, which are legally constituted public bodies, do gain access to personal patient data when it comes to outpatient costs, instead of the insurance organizations, although these establishments are only indirectly involved in patient care.

Generally speaking, the aim should always be to protect the patient's privacy by using anonymous information that can be classified by the use of pseudonyms. But in this connection it should be made clear that with the vast quantity of stored information and the growing integration of databases it is hardly possible any longer to

Figure 14. 3
Flow of Services, Materials and Payments between Service Providers in the Health Insurance System of the Federal Republic of Germany, with Special Emphasis on Compulsory Health Insurance (source German BSI)

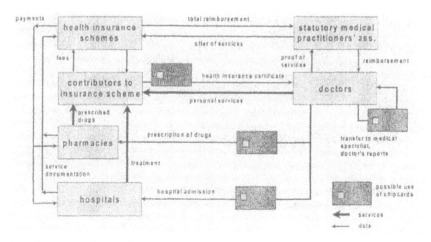

practice anonymity, as the information can be re-identified from the data, that is to say it can be clearly associated with a particular patient.

Consequences for Data Protection and Data Security in Medical Information Systems

Regulations and data protection measures within the health care system contribute to preserving the trust relationship between patient and doctor and the individual rights of the patient during data processing. Data security must be area-specific, especially medicine-specific. In particular, ethical aspects should be included in solutions to the problem of data security in the health care and social welfare services.

Patient data should be protected according to the state of the art, although the principle of relativity should also be observed (cf. EU directive [CE 95]). Medical data with their high sensitivity require a particular effort in order to ensure security. Technical and administrative means must be made available to ensure that doctors and care staff and other authorized persons[9] can read the patient data or pass them on within the permitted context. Even the hospital administration should only have access to the data that are essential for their purposes. As a form of technical security, patient data (and any other possibly confidential data) should be protected at each system set-up against viewing and transmission; giving out any information should be a conscious act. Depending on the various tasks and purposes access should be selectively allowed (CE 95) by:

- identification data;

- administrative data;

- social data;

- medical data;

- genetic data.

Security measures should not distract the attention of the doctor from the patient. It is true that data protection measures cannot take place without the cooperation of the persons involved, but the burden on the medical staff arising from administrative and technical procedures should be kept to a minimum. Correct handling of patient data should not be adversely affected by protection measures. Availability of the data, especially in critical situations, must be guaranteed in the interests of the patient. Availability of the data should also be guaranteed in the justified general interest, although in this case strict criteria must be applied.

Technical data protection measures should present minimum barriers to the exchange of non-sensitive information, for example access to external information services on the Internet or by email. The use of data for research purposes should also be allowed, provided the data protection laws for scientific research projects[2] are respected. The data used in this way should be made anonymous at the earliest opportunity. If the research aim requires data from different sources to be assimilated, or cases to be re-identifiable, pseudonyms should be used. (Pommerening 95).

Technical and administrative data protection measures in a health care establishment should not be treated as a subsidiary task. They require the creation of a suitable infrastructure and clear delineation of responsibilities as well as built-in planning for an appropriate investment of finances and persons.

Systems Models and Implementation of Secure Information Systems

Before setting up an information system, especially bearing in mind the security required by a health care system, there should be a clear definition of the practical aims and the anticipated uses; and problems should be identified and possible solutions put forward. Developing solutions and implementing them fully within the existing application environment requires clear definition of tasks, division of tasks, communication and cooperation between developers/ systems providers, management and users (Blobel 95b). As the IT applications that are introduced must be compatible with the aims and processes of the establishment in question, the most important activity is a clear and comprehensive description of in-house policy (aims; measures; assessment criteria for management, processes and quality.) The second activity should be directed towards the complex analysis of processes, including integration mechanisms (Blobel

95 b; Blobel 96 d). Then there should also be a general risk analysis of the system and its environment along with a definition of threats and countermeasures. Frequently not enough attention is paid to quality management and systems assessment as part of the development result, yet they are particularly important for the success of an information system (EC 91a; SEISMED 96).

In order to develop and implement secure information systems it is essential to allocate and describe responsibilities internally as well as with outside establishments involved. It goes without saying that users should be integrated and staff representatives involved.

All activities must be subject to documentation and detailed protocols in the implementation phase. At each stage of development and implementation it is important to continually update the security rules and raise data security awareness. A very high priority should be given to training, professional qualifications and staff development both of management and workers (SEISMED 96).

The following principles should be observed for the storage, communication and processing of data in health care information systems (Blobel 95 a; Blobel 96 a, b):

- Systems organization including the communication infrastructure (network topology) should take account of structural units and common functional factors/conditions.

- The number of authorized personnel and their rights should always be kept to a minimum.

- The establishment or department that collects the data is responsible for storage and processing and must ensure that it is protected from other establishments or departments. Collecting agents are responsible for the data collected and for the function and access rights to these data. This means that rights can only be allocated to third parties (logical delegation) and may never be assumed by them of their own initiative.

- Production, testing and training must be strictly separated.

- The ISO safety standards for networks must be applied (Ruhland 93; Stallings 95).

The constraints imposed by the concept of security must be guaranteed in the implementation, that is to say security technology must be used to put them into practice. An example is to specify who has access to what information. One should also not overlook the possibilities of data access circumventing the application programs, for example with the aid of direct access to the storage medium or network monitoring programs.

Security Concepts, Services and Mechanisms

In order to realize the concept of data security technically it is useful to structure the security architecture according to functional criteria or needs and to base the data security services on generic data security models. Figure 14.4 shows a layered model of data security, where amongst the general more comprehensive concepts of data security only the concept security is included and the concepts quality and safety are omitted.

Communication and cooperation in health care, and also elsewhere, must take place on the basis of trust. For this reason a basic requirement is mutual and certified strong authentication of the principals involved (this notion includes the human user as well as machines, systems, applications and apparatus). This authentication service is simultaneously required for numerous other security services (authorization, access controls, audit, etc.) The communicated

Figure 14.4
Layered Model of Security Architecture

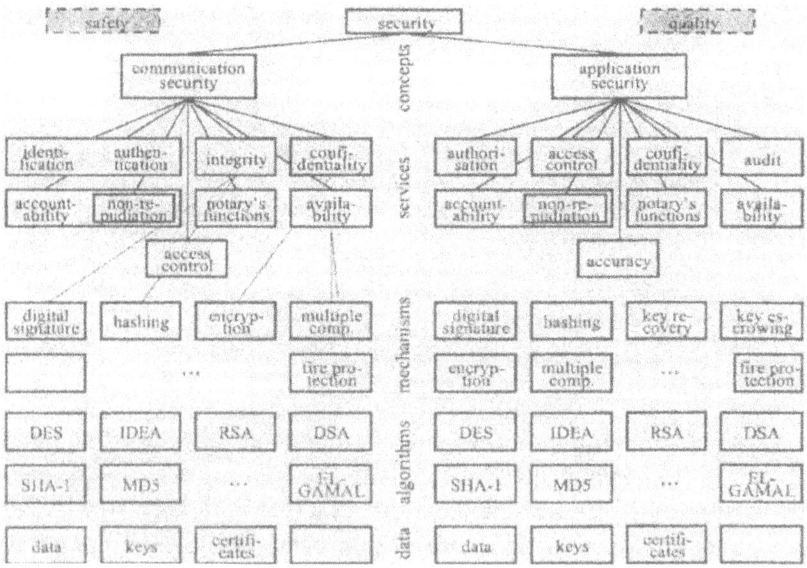

information has to be integer and realized according to the agreed policy (e.g., trustworthy, classified, grouped). Data and processes (functionality) have to be accountable.

This complex concept of security requirements is also called communication security. In order to provide the required services cryptographic mechanisms are used. Basically, there is a distinction between symmetric procedures, where the same secret key is used for encoding and decoding, and asymmetric procedures, which uses different keys for encoding and decoding that belong only to one single pair.[3] Apart from simplifying key distribution and key management, asymmetric procedures use corresponding mechanisms, such as digital signatures, to facilitate specific security services such as authentication of origin and accountability of information (see below). Because the user can receive and send communications from and to different domains (e.g., work-place, department, organization, group) the services and mechanisms involved have to be organized globally or at least within the agreed user domain (data capture area). Included in the common domain are the unified assignment of names and the availability of keys, certificates and certificate revocation lists that are held in directories and updated.

In accordance with the fair information principles and the legal and ethical foundations for health care discussed above, the need-to-know principle and the doctor-patient trust relationship have to be guaranteed. (Kluge 95). By contrast, user authorization for specific information and processes, access to defined information (data) and application functionality and guarantees of their quality and accountability have to be organized within the direct responsibility of the user, originator or administrator of the information, that is, locally. Authorization, access controls, object or document authentication, specification of roles and rules for supporting decisions in access regulations describe the concept of application security and other application-related security services. Details of the analysis and design of secure health care information systems are discussed elsewhere. As these aspects are beyond the scope of this present chapter, the reader is referred to the references (e.g., Blobel 99 a, c, ISHTAR).

Strong authentication of the user, that is, based on cryptographic algorithms, is supported by tokens which within a secure environment contain the private keys (in the case of asymmetric algorithms) or secret keys (in the case of symmetric algorithms) for authentication and other security mechanisms such as digital signature or encryption, and which offer security functions. In Europe and elsewhere smart cards (microprocessor cards with an additional crypto-controller) have been introduced for this purpose. In this way user authentication is ensured not only by internal knowledge, as with a password, but additionally by possession of a token. As this card also contains certified information for health care workers on the structural or functional role of the card holder (Blobel 97 d; Blobel 99 a, c), which can reveal certain rights and obligations, it is also called a Health Professional Card (HPC).

The solutions mentioned above for trustworthy communication and cooperation between health care information systems on the basis of a public key infrastructure (PKI) require independent, trustworthy authorities, so-called trusted third parties (TTP), which confirm allocation of a key to a particular person and that person's role and rights.

National initiatives, such as for example:

- the law on information and communication services (Informations-und Kommunikationdienste-gesetz IuKDG) and related laws (law on digital signature, Signaturgesetz SigG) and the respective rules for application within the Federal Republic of Germany;

- the specifications of the German health professional card (HPC 99a);

- the French regulations for the introduction of the HCP card and for health insurance cards with similar functions for patients, which are discussed in greater detail in another chapter of this volume;

- the Swedish standards for a smart card as a token for strong authentication and digital signature (SS 98);

and standardization on an international level such as:

- the European Electronic Signature Standard Initiative (EESSI) of the European Commission (EC 99); and

- the CEN/TC 251 standard "Health Informatics-secure user identification-strong authentication using microprocessor cards (PT 037 SEC-ID/CARDS)" (CEN 99)

create the conditions for establishing these security services and mechanisms. Apart from that there are system-related security solutions on the Internet such as the secure socket layer (SSL) protocol or the transport layer security (TLS) protocol for secure communication between authentic systems. These protocols do not, however, meet the legal requirements for proof of personal responsibility, so that they should as a rule be used in conjunction with the prescribed person-related mechanisms.

Trustworthy EDI

As explained in the sections above and discussed at length with regard to architectural, data protection and data security requirements, in shared care health care information systems a comprehensive electronic data interchange (EDI) takes place. By means of EDI data with widely varying structures (e.g., results, information on the patient's family, X-rays, invoice details, etc.) are transmitted across networks including the Internet internally and also between health care establishments directly and indirectly involved in patient care (registered doctors, hospitals, university hospitals, pharmacies, health insurance schemes, social services, etc.).

Depending on the operational area, and on the content and use of the information different message definitions, syntax and exchange formats are used. Examples of EDI are the xDT4 and HL75 protocols mentioned above and also medicine-related EDIFACT6 messages and the DICOM standard7 for the communication of images. Because of its universality and optimization in the Internet environment the XML standard is at present being massively promoted. Because of its aptness for message definition; for description, storage and retrieval of complex documents; for communication of documents (exchange format) and for describing user interfaces it will in the medium term replace the other EDI protocols, with the possible exception of the DICOM standards relating especially to channel security.

Because of the sensitivity of patient-related medical data there are very stringent legal and technical requirements to guarantee adequate data security during information exchange between unprotected networks, in particular for the patient but also for health care workers and for the establishments involved. These requirements are met by security services such as identification and strong authentication of the users or computers involved, data confidentiality, data origin authentication, data integrity and accountability in the sense of non-repudiation of origin and receipt.

For communication security both end-to-end security via message wrapping (message security) at the application layer of the ISO-OSI model of communication, and channel security at the lower layers are included in the solutions.

Channel security based solutions are generally transparent for the user and independent of the characteristics of the information transmitted. The security solution based on message security (object security) can also be specified independent of the exchange format of the message transmitted, of the communication protocol and of the cryptographic syntax.

Within the context of the MEDSEC project sponsored by the European Commission (MEDSEC) an open solution has been specified and implemented which relies solely on the available ISO, IETF and NIST standards and connects to the current standardization projects of HL7 and CEN (Blobel 98 c, d).

As already mentioned, a specific security solution is independent of the exchange format of the message to be transmitted (e.g., xDT, HL7, XML), of the communication protocol used (e.g., FTP, e-mail) and of the cryptographic syntax (e.g., S/MIME, PKCS#7). Cryptographic procedures are applied in the interests of communication security to the whole message (message wrapping).

The communication protocol itself is also protected. Account is also taken of the event-driven generation of messages and information exchange through user interaction. For this reason implementation of the European security infrastructure on the basis of health professional cards and related trusted third party services was integrated as an essential component. The protocols used and the services realized make the solutions especially apt for the security of communication with cost units described above.

The functionality of the communication server including the EDI interfaces as adapters for the various syntax formats, semantics and protocols of the proprietary uses can be extended to the cryptographic protocols, services and mechanisms, so that this aspect of secure communication also remains transparent both for the user and the applications developer. The latter merely has to implement an accepted standard. The communication server understands and transmits various protocols. Negotiation of the protocol as part of the policy is supported by a tag-length-value (TLV) mechanism along the lines of XML.

The technical standards discussed here and solutions based on IT security criteria (BSI 95; EC 91 b; ZSI 89) offer the conditions for the creation of trustworthy shared care health care information systems. A major contribution to the realization of the necessary infrastructure is at present being made by the EU Trustworthy Health Telematics project (TrustHealth, TH) and by the multimedia law complex (DB 96).

Responsibility and Organizational Measures

Every establishment in the health care service needs a data protection officer and an IT security officer. These duties must be separate, as the data protection officer acts as a controlling authority and cannot simultaneously do the work. Both functions require, regardless of the size and structure of the establishment, adequate time, means (including space) and support in order to carry out their duties, especially secretarial help for correspondence, documentation and administrative duties. They also need the authority to put their decisions into effect. The duties of the data protection officer are prescribed in the relevant data protection law; he should if possible be qualified in medicine, but law is also appropriate. In detail his duties are:

- documentation of person-related data banks;

- checking and inspecting information systems;

- monitoring, follow-up and assessment of data protection violations;

- target group oriented information and training in data protection issues; advising the various departments;

- assistance in requests for information and at complaints procedures;

- collaboration with the IT security officer;

- representation of the establishment to supervisory bodies and other relevant committees;

- initiation of policy definition including definition of roles and regulations to guarantee data protection and data security in communications and applications.

The IT security officer should be a specialist in computing or medical computing. His job is to set up the data protection and IT security concept for the establishment, to agree it with the data protection officer, to implement it with the help of the available IT personnel and to update it (EC 91 a; SEISMED 96). In detail he is responsible for:

- the physical safety of the computers, networks and data storage media including protection against fire and natural disasters;

- control of data archive security;

- configuration of systems to meet the requirements of the security concept (especially with regard to setting up access rights) (Blobel 95 a, b; Blobel 96 a-e; Seelos 91);

- monitoring the local network for undesirable data flows, especially for unauthorized connections to the Internet (via modems) (Stallings 95);

- management of security passes, passwords and keys (with system support) (Pommerening 91; EC 91 a; SEISMED 96);

- assessment of security-related system records (where necessary raise the alarm and introduce protective measures);

- monitoring the implementation of software;

- checking system installation settings for gaps in security;

- training IT personnel and users in security matters;

- drawing up obligation guidelines for IT personnel and users (in liaison with the data protection officer and the personnel officer) (Seelos 91); and

- technical advice to the data protection officer.

In big organizations such as university hospitals, insurance companies or similar the duties of the data protection officer and the IT security officer each warrant a full post, although the duties of the latter could be distributed amongst several people. Additional support from the available IT personnel is in any event necessary. Furthermore, each department should have its own IT personnel and IT security officer (part-time member of IT personnel) as well as a data protection officer (medical practitioner, also part-time).

In small organizations there is a problem of outsourcing as they need to hire an external security officer. But in this case the responsibility should in all events remain within the establishment, along with adequate basic knowledge of problems and solutions. In the case of the data protection officer it would be sensible to consider appointing one data protection officer to work in several establishments. Because detailed knowledge of local relationships is important, outsourcing is often regarded as ineffective and too expensive.

Recommended Technical Measures and Security Infrastructure

The growing trend, even in larger establishments, to buy in ready-made IT systems and make extensive use of standard software leads to increasing dependence on the manufacturers of these systems, but security has to be taken into account right at the start of conception and development of a system and cannot as a rule be satisfactorily grafted onto a ready-made system (EC 91a; SEISMED 96). The systems available at the present time at best fulfil one or two of the essential criteria for open systems listed below:

- encrypted data storage;

- encrypted communication (data transmission);

- checkable access controls (mandatory) on the basis of an access matrix defined for the whole system with decentralized responsibility for access rights (Blobel 96 d; Seelos 91);

- management and control of access to sensitive information in the course of care using authorization by the data protection officer in line with the policy, the roles and the rules that apply to them (discretionary) (Blobel 96 d);

- accountability and integrity of prescriptions, requests for services, communication and documentation using electronic signatures;

- setting up the technical criteria for integrating the future health professional card and establishing the necessary trustworthy key management infrastructure to go with it (trusted authorities, trusted third parties and secure communication with them) (AK 96; Blobel 96 a, b; CEN 99; HPC 99 a; TH);

- integration of PC and network security systems, and

- secure Internet connection using a firewall system (Chapman 95; CTR 96; Stallings 95).

There is in fact rapid technical progress at the present time towards the realization of these criteria. One can only appeal to the manufacturers not to slow down this development and in particular to acquire the cryptographic know-how as fast as possible. Those responsible for the purchase of IT systems in health care should insist that manufacturers and retailers fulfil the above list of criteria.

The technical systems should be easy to understand and transparent for the user and should not overload the user with complicated procedures; they should make it possible to monitor the values which underpin the usefulness of the data. The user should not, however, be able to switch them off at will or to circumvent them.

Conclusions and Perspectives

The current open information systems do not guarantee the necessary level of data protection and data security for use in the health care system. The technical means are, however, available to integrate these into the public health insurance systems at no great additional cost: microchip card readers are widely available and their specifications in the interests of data protection and data security are defined (AG 95), the health professional card is being tested in the field (AK 96; Blobel 99 b) and cryptographic software is freely available (Schneier 96).

From the user's point of view, significant technical security measures do not necessarily mean that there will be hindrances in work processes. But the measures recommended above do require considerable organizational effort. This will lead to a major improvement in the quality of information data and to fulfilling the legal requirements. The costs that arise from this exercise are easily taken up by the rationalizing effect of information technology within the health care system.

Communication of person-related medical data, in particular as far as establishments not directly involved in the health care of the patient are concerned, has to be handled with the greatest care and sensitivity observing the exact and restrictive conditions set by the legal guidelines. The basic principles of data protection and data security described in this chapter such as the need-to-know principle, the principle of minimum rights, earliest possible deletion of data or earliest possible anonymity of information have a particularly high priority in this area, which also includes the health insurance schemes. As has been rightly said by the president of AOK Schleswig-Holstein, data protection and data security should no longer be seen as a burdensome nuisance, but as a major part of service to the client. Data protection and observing professional secrecy within the social services become just as important as for example a proper and up-to-date benefits service.

Data protection and data security demand knowledge, qualifications and professional training in everyone involved, from managers through IT personnel to the user, including the patient. They also require organization and technical means.

The time is ripe to make a serious effort to improve data protection and data security in information systems.

Notes

1. Strafgesetzbuch = Penal Code.
2. Bundesdatenschutzgesetz = Federal data protection law.
3. Health Level 7, a protocol for systems-free data communication in health care (www.hl7.org).
4. Series of standards for communication between surgery computer systems and between them and other service providers of primary care in Germany, coordinated by the Central Research Institute for Ambulatory Care (Zentralinstitut der Kassenärztlichen Bundesvereinigung ZI).
5. Extensible Markup Language: Internet based standard for the definition, description, communication and storage of files, separate description of their composition and management (data retrieval).
6. Common object broker architecture is the object-oriented architecture of an object management group (OMG) for distributed co-operating information systems (www.omg.org).
7. Architecture of interoperable components by Microsoft (DCOM = Distributed component object model).
8. Distributed Health Care Environment describes the European architecture for health care information systems and their standardization (for references cf. (Blobel 97c).
9. According to the EU directive (CE 95) all persons who in the context of their activity have access to personal data are bound to secrecy regardless of whether such an oath exists in their profession or not.
10. §40 BDSG cf. (DSKRP 87).
11. Asymmetric cryptographic procedures are based on the use of pairs of keys, where there is a unique key for the sole use of the key holder, in this case the card holder,

and another key that is made generally available via public directories. Information that is encoded with one key can be decoded with the other key in the pair, which is how the various security services and mechanisms work.

12. Also called data storage media and used for special purposes in primary care, e.g. invoice data, treatment data, laboratory data or instrument data storage.

13. Originally developed for communication within a hospital, but since extended to the whole health care system.

14. EDI for administration, commerce and transport, universal within the framework of the UN-managed EDI format.

15. Digital image communication, advanced by the DICOM Working Group of the American College of Radiology and the National Electrical Manufacturers Association.

References

(AG 95)   Arbeitsgemeinschaft "Karten im Gesundheitswesen," GMD-Forschungszentrum Informationstechnik GmbH (1995) Multifunktionale KartenTerminals (MKT) für das Gesundheitswesen und andere Anwendungsgebiete. Spezifikation Version 1.0, August 1995.

(AK 96)   Arbeitskreis "Health Professional Card" der Arbeitsgemeinschaft "Karten im Gesundheitswesen" (1996) Deutscher Modellversuch "Health Professional Card (HPC)," Göttingen, Oktober 1996.

(ASTM E 1869)   Standard Guide for Confidentiality, Privacy, Access, and Data Security Principles for Health Information Including Computer-Based Patient Records. Annual Book of ASTM Standards, Vol. 14.01.

(ASTM PS 101)   Provisional Guide on Security Framework for Health Care Information. Annual Book of ASTM Standards, Vol. 14.01.

(ASTM PS 108)   Provisional Guide for Individual Rights Regarding Health Information. Annual Book of ASTM Standards, Vol. 14.01.

(Bakker 95)   Bakker, A.R., et al. (Edrs.) (1995) Caring for Health Information. Safety, Security and Secrecy. North-Holland, Amsterdam.

(Barber 96)   Barber B., Treacher A., and Louwerse K. (eds.) (1996) Towards Security in Medical Telematics. Series in Health Technology and Informatics Vol. 27. IOS Press, Amsterdam.

(BfD 95)   Der Bundesbeauftragte für den Datenschutz (1995) 15. Tätigkeitsbericht 1993-1994 (Barber96).

(Blobel 95a)   Blobel, B. (Hrg.) (1995) Datenschutz in medizinischen Informationssystemen. Vieweg, Braunschweig, Wiesbaden.

(Blobel 95b)   Blobel, B. (1995) GSG '93 und GNG '95—Umstrukturierung der Krankenhaussysteme. klinikarzt Nr. 10/24 (1995) 491-499.

(Blobel 96a)   Blobel, B. (1995) Clinical Record Systems in Oncology. Experiences and Developments on Cancer Registries in Eastern Germany, in Preproceedings of the International Workshop "Personal Information—Security, Engineering and Ethics" pp. 37-54, Cambridge, 21-22 June, 1996, also published in R. Anderson (Edr.) Personal Medical Information—Security, Engineering, and Ethics, pp. 39-56. Spinger, Berlin, New York 1997.

(Blobel 96b)   Blobel, B. (1996) A Regional Clinical Cancer Documentation System for an Optimal Shared Health Care in Cancer, in Medical Informatics Europe '96 (eds. J. Brender, J. P. Christensen, J.-R. Scherrer, P. McNair), pp. 1019-1026. IOS Press, Amsterdam.

(Blobel 96c)   Blobel, B. (1996) Datensicherheit in offenen Gesundheits-
                informationssystemen, Teil 1. krankenhausumschau 11, S. 852-857.
(Blobel 96d)   Blobel, B. (1996) Datensicherheit in offenen Gesundheits-
                informationssystemen, Teil 2. krankenhausumschau 12, S. 934-937.
(Blobel 96e)   Blobel, B. (1996) Datensicherheitsaspekte beim standardisierten
                Datenaustausch im Gesundheitswesen. In Mayr, H. T., Informatik '96.
                Beherrschung von Informationssystemen, Band 8, S. 155-165. R.
                Oldenbourg Verlag, München und Wien.
(Blobel 96d)   Blobel, B. (1996) Modelling for Design and Implementation of Secure
                Health Information Systems. International Journal of Bio-Medical Com-
                puting 43, S23-S30.
(Blobel 97a)   Blobel B. (1997) Security requirements and solutions in distributed
                Electronic Health Records, in Information Security in Research and
                Business (eds. L. Yngström, and J. Carlsen), pp. 377-390. Chapman &
                Hall, London.
(Blobel 97b)   Blobel B., Bleumer G., Müller A., Flikkenschild E., and Ottes F. (1997)
                Current Security Issues Faced by Health Care Establishments. Deliver-
                able of the HC1028 Telematics Project ISHTAR, February 1997.
(Blobel 97c)   Blobel, B., Holena, M. (1997) Comparing middleware concepts for
                advanced health care system architectures. International Journal of
                Medical Informatics 46, pp. 69-85 .
(Blobel 97d)   Blobel, B., Pharow, P. (1997) Security Infrastructure of an Oncological
                Network Using Health Professional Cards, in Health Cards '97 (eds. L.
                van den Broek, A.J. Sikkel) , pp. 323-334. Series in Health Technology
                and Informatics Vol. 49. IOS Press, Amsterdam.
(Blobel 98a)   Blobel, B., Holena, M. (1998) CORBA Security Services for Health
                Information Systems. International Journal of Medical Informatics 52
                1-3, pp. 29-38.
(Blobel 98b)   Blobel, B., Katsikas, S.K. (1998) Patient data and the Internet—secu-
                rity issues. Chairpersons' introduction. International Journal of Medi-
                cal Informatics 49, pp. S5-S8.
(Blobel 98c)   Blobel, B., Spiegel, V., Krohn, R., Pharow, P., Engel, K. (1998) Stan-
                dard Guide for HL7 Communication Security. ISIS MEDSEC Project,
                Deliverable 30, August 1998.
(Blobel 98d)   Blobel, B., Spiegel, V., Krohn, R., Pharow, P., Engel, K. (1998) Stan-
                dard Guide for Implementing EDI Communication Security. ISIS
                MEDSEC Project, Deliverable 31, August 1998.
(Blobel 99a)   Blobel, B., Pharow, P., Roger-France, F. (1999) Security Analysis and
                Design Based on a General Conceptual Security Model and UML, in
                High Performance Computing and Networking (eds. P. Sloot, M. Bubak,
                A. Hoekstra, B. Hertzberger), pp. 919-930. Lecture Notes in Computer
                Sciences 1593. Springer, Berlin, Heidelberg, New York.
(Blobel 99b)   Blobel, B., and Pharow, P. (1999) Secure Communications and Co-
                operations in Open Networks, in Recent Advances in Signal Process-
                ing and Communications (ed. N.E. Mastorakis), pp. 356-362. World
                Scientific and Engineering Society Press.
(Blobel 99c)   Blobel, B, Roger-France, F., Pharow, P. (1999) A Systematic Approach
                for Secure Health Information Systems. International Journal of Medi-
                cal Informatics.
(BSI 95)   Bundesamt für Sicherheit in der Informationstechnik: IT-
                Grundschutzhandbuch- - Massnahmenempfehlung für den mittleren

Schutzbedarf. Schriftenreihe zur IT Sicherheit, Bundesanzeiger Verlag GmbH, 1995, Germany.

(CE 95)   Council of Europe (1995) Directive 95/46/EC on the Protection of Individuals with Regard to the Processing of Personal Data and on the Free Movement of such Data. Strasbourg.

(CEN 99)   CEN TC 251 (1999) PT37: Health Informatics—Secure User Identification-Strong Authentication using Microprocessor Cards (SEC-ID/CARDS).

(CERT)   CERT Co-ordination Centre, http://www.cert.org.

(Chapman 95)   Chapman, D. B., and Zwicky, Elizabeth D. (1995) Building Internet Firewalls. O'Reilly Associates, Inc., Sebastopol.

(CM 97)   Committee of Ministers (1997) European Recommendation (Draft) No. R(96) of the Committee of Ministers to Member States on the Protection of Medical Data (and Genetic Data). CJ-PD (96). Strasbourg.

(CoA 88)   Commonwealth of Australia (1988) Privacy Act No. 119, Canberra.

(CTR 96)   CTR (1996) Security Issues for the Internet and the World Wide Web; CTR Report No 8, Computer Technology Research Corp., Charleston.

(DSKRP 87)   Datenschutzkommission Rheinland-Pfalz, Mainz (1987) Datenschutzrechtliche Anforderungen an wissenschaftlichen Forschungsvorhaben, Mainz.

(DB 96)   Der Deutsche Bundestag (1996) Multimedia-Gesetz (Referenten-Entwurf) Bonn, 1996.
http://www.uni-duesseldorf.de/WWW/Jura/internet/netlaw/IuKDG.htm
1) Gesetz zur Regelung der Rahmenbedingungen für Informations-und Kommunikationsdienste (Information-und Kommunikationsdienste-Gesetz-IuKDG) in der Fassung des Beschlusses des Deutschen Bundestages vom 13. Juni 1997 (BT-Drs. 13/7934 vom 11.06.1997).
2.) Katalog der technischen Fragen zum Thema: Anforderungen an die Infrastruktur bei der Implementierung der digitalen Signatur, 20.3.1997
3) Maßnahmenkataloge zur digitalen Signatur, 1.7.1997
4) Chipkarten als Signaturkomponente, Maßnahmenkatalog, 26.5.1997.

(EC 91a)   The Commission of the European Communities DG XIII/F AIM (1991) Data Protection and Confidentiality in Health Informatics, AIM Working Conference, Brussels, 19-21 March 1990, IOS Press, Amsterdam, Washington DC, Tokio.

(EC 91b)   European Communities-Commission: ITSEC: Information Technology Security Evaluation Criteria; (Provisional Harmonised Criteria, Version 1.2, 28 June 1991). Office for Official Publications of the European Communities, Luxembourg 1991.

(EC 99)   European Communities-Commission (1999) European Electronic Signature Standard Initiative (EESSI).

(Ellsässer 93)   Ellsässer, K.-H., Köhler, C.O. Shared Care: Konzept einer verteilten Pflege-Kurz-und langfristige Perspektiven in Europa. Informatik, Biometrie und Epidemiologie in Medizin und Biologie 24 (1993) H.4, S. 188-198.

(EUROMED)   The EUROMED-ETS Consortium. EUROMED-European Trust Structure. Information Society Standardisation Programme. http://

euromed.iccs.ntua.gr/.

(HPC 99a)   HPC Specification Final German version 1.0 of the Specification of the German Doctors' Licence including the Specification of related Certificates (1999) http://www.hcp-protocol.de/arztausw/ arztausw.htm.

(HPC 99b)   HPC Specification English Draft version 0.9 of the Specification of the German Doctors' Licence including the Specification of related Certificates (1999). http://www.hcp-protocol.de/arztausw/ engausw.htm.

(ISHT)   The ISHTAR Consortium. Implementation of Secure Health Telematics Applications in Europe. Project of the Fourth EU Health Telematics Applications Programme. http://ted.see.plym.ac.uk/ ishtar/

(Kluge 95)   E.-H. W. Kluge: Patients, Patient Records, and Ethical Principles. In: R. A. Green et al. (Edrs.): MEDINFO '95, pp. 1596-1600. Noth-Holland, Amsterdam-London-New York-Tokyo 1995 .

(Katsikas 98)   Katsikas, S. K., Spinellis, D. D., Iliadis, J., Blobel, B. (1998) Using Trusted Third Parties for secure telemedical applications over the WWW: The EUROMED-ETS approach. International Journal of Medical Informatics 49, pp. 59-68.

(LDSH 99)   Der Landesbeauftragte für den Datenschutz Schleswig-Holstein (1999) 21. Tätigkeitsbericht 1999.

(MEDSEC)   MEDSEC Consortium, Health Care Security and Privacy in the Information Society. Project of the EU ISIS Programme. http:// www.math.aegean.gr/info-sec/projects/medsec.htm.

(McCurley 95)   McCurley, K.S. (1995) Protecting privacy and information integrity of computerised medical information. http://www.cs.sandia.gov/ ~mccurley/health.html.

(Pommerening 91) Pommerening, K. (1991) Datenschutz und Datensicherheit. BI-Wissenschaftsverlag, Mannheim, Wien, Zürich.

(Pommerening 95) Pommerening, K. (1995) Pseudonyme-ein Kompromiß zwischen Anonymisierung und Personenbezug, in Medizinische Forschung-ärztliches Handeln (Hrg. H.J. Trampisch, S. Lange,), S. 329-333. MMV Medizin Verlag, München.

(Ruhland 93)   Ruhland, Ch. (1993) Informationssicherheit in Datennetzen. DATACOM-Verlag.

(Schneier 96)   Schneier, B. (1996) Applied Cryptography. Second Edition. John Wiley & Sons, Inc., New York.

(Seelos 91)   Seelos, H-J. (1991) Informationssysteme und Datenschutz im Krankenhaus. DuD-Fachbeiträge 14. Vieweg, Braunschweig, Wiesbaden.

(SS 98)   Swedish Standard 62 43 30 (1998) Identification Cards—Electronic ID Application.

(Stallings95)   Stallings, W. (1995) Network and Internet Security. Principles and Practice. Prentice Hall, Hemel Hempstead.

(SEISMED 96)   The SEISMED Consortium, (edr.) (1996) Data Security for Health Care. Volume I-III. Studies in Health Technology and Informatics, Vol. 31-33. IOS Press, Amsterdam.

(TH)   The TrustHealth Consortium. Trustworthy Health Telematics 1. Project of the Fourth EU Health Telematics Applications Programme. http:// www.ramit.be/trusthealth http://www.spri.se/th2/default.htm.

(USC 74)   U.S. Congress (1974) Privacy Act of 1974, USC 552a Public Law 93-079.

(USC 96)   U.S. Congress (1996) The Health insurance Portability and Account-
              ability Act of 1996, Public Law 104-191.
(ZSI 89)   Zentralstelle für Sicherheit in der Informationstechnik, Köln (1989)
              IT-Sicherheitskriterien - Kriterien für die Bewertung der Sicherheit
              von Systemen der Informationstechnik (IT), Köln.

Contributors

Bernd Blobel

Otto-von-Guericke University Magdeburg
Head of Department
Department of Medical Informatics
Leipziger Str. 44,
DE-39210 Magdeburg
Germany

Gerhard Brenner

Central Research Institute of Ambulatory Health
Care
Secretary
Herbert-Lewin Strasse 5
DE - 50931 Cologne
Germany

Claude Delaveau

Primary Health Fund
Director General
195 avenue Paul-Vailland Couturier
FR - 93014 Bobigny Cedex
France

Maurice Duranton

National Federation of Public Service Mutual
Benefit Societies
President
17 avenue de Choisy
FR - 75640 Paris
France

Rena Eichler

Management Science for Health
Health Reform and Financing Program
Senior Health Economist
165 Allandale Road
Boston, MA 02130
USA

Wouter van Ginneken   International Labour Office
                           Social Security Department
                           Senior Economist
                           Route des Morillons 4
                           CH - 1211 Geneva 22
                           Switzerland

Navin Girishankar   World Bank
                           Operations Evaluation Department
                           Evaluation Officer
                           1818 H Street, N.W.
                           Washington, DC 20433
                           USA

Thomas Hansmeier   Humboldt University Berlin
                           Institute for Rehabilitation
                           Research Assistant
                           Luisenstr. 13 a
                           DE - 10098 Berlin
                           Germany

April Harding   World Bank
                           Private Sector Development Department
                           Private Sector Development Specialist
                           1818 H Street, N.W.
                           Washington, DC 20433
                           USA

Aidi Hu   International Labour Office
                           Social Security Specialist
                           Route des Morillons 4
                           CH - 1211 Geneva 22
                           Switzerland

Naoki Iguchi   Ministry of Health and Welfare
                           Health and Welfare Bureau for the Elderly
                           Director of Planning Division
                           1-2-2, Kasumigaseki, Chiyoda-ku
                           Tokyo 100-8045
                           Japan

Werner Müller-Fahrnow   Humboldt University Berlin
                         Institute for Rehabilitation
                         Professor
                         Luisenstr. 13 a
                         DE - 10098 Berlin
                         Germany

William Newbrander   Management Science for Health
                         Health Reform and Financing Program
                         Director
                         165 Allandale Road
                         Boston, MA 02130
                         USA

Julio Pilón   Union of Mutual Benefit Societies of Uruguay
                         Tresorer
                         Paysandú 941 Piso 6 of 4
                         UY - 11.100 Montevideo
                         Uruguay

Alexander Preker   World Bank
                         Health, Nutrition, and Population Department
                         Lead Economist
                         1818 H Street, N.W.
                         Washington, DC 20433
                         USA

Aviva Ron   World Health Organization
                         Health Infrastructure
                         Director
                         Western Pacific Regional Office
                         P.O. Box 2932 (United Nations Ave.)
                         1000 Manila
                         Philippines

Xenia Scheil-Adlung   International Social Security Association
                         Studies and Operations Branch
                         Program Manager
                         Case postale 1
                         CH - 1211 Geneva 22

Karla Spyra   Humboldt University Berlin
                               Institute for Rehabilitation
                               Research Assistant
                               Luisenstr. 13 a
                               DE - 10098 Berlin
                               Germany

Abdellatif Zuaq   National Fund of Social Insurance Organiza-
                               tions
                               Director
                               B.P. 209
                               8, rue Al Khalil
                               MA - Rabat
                               Maroc

Index